ESSAYS ON

SOME MALADIES OF ANGOLA

(1799)

ENSAIOS

SOBRE

ALGUMAS ENFERMIDADES

D'ANGOLA,

DEDICADOS

AO

SERENISSIMO SENHOR

D. JOÃO

PRINCIPE DO BRAZIL

POR

JOSE' PINTO DE AZEREDO,

Cavalleiro da Ordem de Christo, Doutor em Medicina, e Socio de varias Academias da Europa.

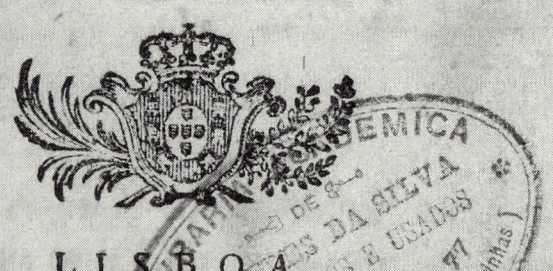

LISBOA,

NA REGIA OFFICINA TYPOGRAFICA

M. DCC. XCIX.

Com licença da Meza do Desembargo da Paço.

ESSAYS ON

SOME MALADIES OF ANGOLA

(1799)

José Pinto de Azeredo

Translated by Stewart Lloyd-Jones

EDITED BY

TIMOTHY D. WALKER

ADELINO CARDOSO

ANTÓNIO BRAZ DE OLIVEIRA

MANUEL SILVÉRIO MARQUES

Tagus Press | *UMass Dartmouth*

DARTMOUTH, MASSACHUSETTS

*Tagus Press is the publishing arm of the
Center for Portuguese Studies and Culture at
the University of Massachusetts Dartmouth.*
Center Director: João M. Paraskeva

Classic Histories from the Portuguese-Speaking World in Translation 2
SERIES EDITORS: Timothy J. Coates and Timothy D. Walker

Tagus Press at UMass Dartmouth
www.portstudies.umassd.edu
© 2016 The University of Massachusetts Dartmouth
Managing Editor: Mario Pereira
Copyedited by Glenn E. Novak
Designed by April Leidig
Typeset in Caslon by Copperline Book Services, Inc.

For all inquiries, please contact:
Tagus Press • Center for Portuguese Studies and Culture
UMass Dartmouth • 285 Old Westport Road
North Dartmouth MA 02747-2300
Tel. 508-999-8255 • Fax 508-999-9272
www.portstudies.umassd.edu

Paperback: ISBN 978-1-933227-69-6 | Ebook: ISBN 978-1-933227-70-2

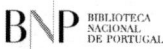 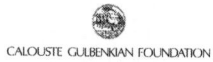 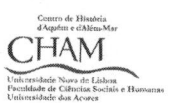 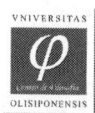

This work was published with the support of the Fundação Calouste Gulbenkian,
the Centro de História da Cultura/Centro de História d'Além Mar at the
Universidade Nova de Lisboa, the Centro de Filosofia at the Universidade de
Lisboa, and the Biblioteca Nacional de Portugal.

5 4 3 2 1

FRONTIS: Title page from José Pinto de Azeredo, *Ensaios sobre algumas
enfermidades de Angola*, Lisbon, 1799; original at the John Carter Brown Library,
Providence, Rhode Island. Courtesy of the John Carter Brown Library at
Brown University.

CONTENTS

Early modern and Enlightenment-era medical texts are notoriously difficult to translate for presentation to a modern audience. Produced at a time when concepts of healing—and ideas about observing, recording, and interpreting the natural world—were in profound transition, and when standardized scientific methods of describing phenomena were in their infancy, such texts present distinct editorial challenges in effectively conveying their complexity and richness. One must interpret not only linguistic differences, but also bridge a cosmological gap, presenting a premodern worldview in a way that is intelligible to modern readers whose outlook, at least toward health and healing, is shaped wholly by contemporary medical science. The editorial team has worked closely with the translator, Stewart Lloyd-Jones, in an attempt to convey the important content of Azeredo's text, along with its unique tone and spirit derived from the chronological and geographical context in which the work was originally composed.

In many instances, Azeredo's specific contemporary medical terms are profoundly difficult to render accurately in contemporary English —either the cognate has fallen into disuse, changed in meaning, or lost resonance to our modern ear. Often employing a more precise, historically accurate translated term is not the best option, because the modern reader is not likely to understand, or the word does not convey meaning clearly. In such cases, I have often inserted a more apt or recognizable term, or added a clarifying footnote. For example, even though the translated terms are anachronistic, for our purposes "temperature" works better in English than Azeredo's original term, "body heat," and "pulse" is clearer than "heartbeat." Similarly, we chose to alter Azeredo's original title, because in English the word "maladies" more precisely captures the meaning of the Portuguese word *enfermidades* than does the English cognate, "infirmities."

In general, Portuguese names for people have been given in their modern form; place names have been given in the form most commonly accepted in Anglophone usage. The translation of names for medical substances and medicinal plants often presented a challenge, for two reasons: imprecision in contemporary eighteenth-century nomenclature often creates doubt regarding the precise plant or substance Azeredo referred to in the text, and sometimes indigenous plant names in the Lusophone world have no specific English equivalent. In such cases, an editorial note has been introduced to clarify the matter.

For the readers' convenience, the use of non-English and technical words is limited in this book, except in cases where use of specific vocabulary helps to highlight contemporary medical methodologies, or cultural circumstances. When unfamiliar terms or persons required a brief historical footnote to orient the modern reader, these have been provided. The guiding principle, of course, was to transform a highly technical historical text, brimming with cultural and scientific complexities, into a readable and edifying tool for modern students, especially undergraduates with little or no training in medical history.

Timothy D. Walker
New Bedford, Massachusetts
25 June 2015

ACKNOWLEDGMENTS

A project of this scale and broad topical scope can best be brought to fruition through collaborative means; we therefore assembled a team of highly experienced medical historians whose collective strengths, skills, and scholarly activities promised a highly interdisciplinary and multifaceted approach to this volume. I would first like to thank my colleagues in Portugal, coeditors Adelino Cardoso, Manuel Silvério Marques, and António Braz de Oliveira, for bringing this project to my attention, inviting me to participate as the editor of the Tagus Press volume, and trusting to my editorial instincts in creating this first English edition of José Pinto de Azeredo's work. We all share a profound gratitude to the Fundação Calouste Gulbenkian, and to the Centro de História da Cultura—now amalgamated with the Centro de História d'Aquém e d'Além-Mar (CHAM)—Universidade Nova de Lisboa, for their generous donations supporting the translation of this volume. Our sincere thanks go to Stewart Lloyd-Jones, director of the Contemporary Portuguese History Research Centre (CPHRC), for his exemplary and dedicated work on the translation. We would also like to extend our thanks to Dr. Timothy Coates, coeditor of the Tagus Press series Classic Histories from the Portuguese-Speaking World in Translation, for his critical reading of the introductory essays and main text. To Mario Pereira, managing editor of Tagus Press, we offer our thanks for his assistance in shepherding the project through all its stages, from development to publication. We would also like to acknowledge the important assistance and contributions made to this work by Professor Laurinda Abreu of the Universidade de Évora; Teresa Saraiva and Isabel Abecasis of the Torre do Tombo, the Portuguese National Archive; by the staffs of the National Library of Portugal and the Oporto Municipal Public Library (especially Dr. Júlio Rodrigues da Costa); and by the physicians João David de Morais, Joaquim Barradas, and Pedro Abecasis. In particular, I would like to offer my personal gratitude to Manuel Marques as the original impetus behind this edition, and António Braz de Oliveira for his critical reading of the translated text, and for his many suggestions for editorial revisions that ultimately have made this text far stronger. Finally, for the exceptional aid they provided in the preparation of this volume, I would like to draw attention to three new works of scholarship about Azeredo's life and works that have been published recently in Portugal by the coeditors of this volume. I am confident that these Portuguese-language editions will be recognized as the definitive treatments of Azeredo's achievement in medical science during the late eighteenth century. A new annotated edition of *Ensaios sobre algumas enfermidades de Angola*, edited by António Braz de Oliveira and Manuel Silvério Marques, was published in Lisbon by Colibri Press in 2013. The following year, Colibri published a critical edition of José Pinto de Azeredo's *Isagòge pathologica do corpo humano*, again edited by António Braz de Oliveira and Manuel Silvério Marques. Also in 2014, Colibri published José Pinto de Azeredo's *Tratado anatómico dos ossos, vasos lymphaticos e glândulas*, edited by Júlio Rodrigues da Costa, in collaboration with António Braz de Oliveira, Manuel Silvério Marques, and Paula Andrade Martins. A fourth publication, a critical edition of Azeredo's work titled *Colecção de observações clínicas* is on the way, currently being produced by our colleagues in Brazil: André Luís Lima Nogueira (who did the transcriptions), in collaboration with Jean Luiz Abreu, Junia Furtado, and Valéria Mara. We are very grateful for their work.

Timothy D. Walker
New Bedford, Massachusetts
25 June 2015

ESSAYS ON

SOME MALADIES OF ANGOLA

(1799)

Medical Inquiry in the Enlightenment-Era Portuguese Imperial World

Azeredo's Scientific Publications in Context

Timothy D. Walker

(University of Massachusetts–Dartmouth)

When José Pinto de Azeredo composed and published "Chemical Examination of the Atmosphere of Rio de Janeiro" (*Jornal Enciclopédico*, Lisbon, 1790) and *Essays on Some Maladies of Angola* (Lisbon, 1799), he contributed quite deliberately and consciously to an ongoing scientific conversation with a learned European community whose empirical aspirations had long achieved a global reach, especially in regard to medicine. This broad vision toward addressing matters of health with newfound tropical remedies grew in no small part from maritime exploration and colonization initiated by the Portuguese in the early fifteenth century.[1] Azeredo, born in Brazil in 1764 into an intellectual environment marginalized by distance from European centers of learning and fettered by the restrictive policies of the Portuguese Overseas Council[2] and the Inquisition Censorship Board,[3] first had the opportunity to fully appreciate and engage in this international exchange of ideas while pursuing his medical studies in northern Europe as a very young man.

Azeredo's life and work exemplify two trends distinguishable in Portuguese medical history during the long eighteenth century. First, Azeredo followed a path of many Lusophone physicians before him who sought training with well-known innovative medical practitioners in northern Europe—in France, England, Scotland, and the Netherlands. Second, Azeredo's publications should be understood in context as part of an Enlightenment-era effort by Portuguese authorities to gather strategic medical information from throughout the Lusophone world in a comprehensive attempt to improve imperial health conditions, thereby protecting their comparatively modest and vulnerable human resources. Thus, this effort emerged as a centrally directed policy intended to support the entire colonial enterprise.

Across western Europe, the rhythm of state-supported scientific missions overseas ticked up after the mid-eighteenth century, with European government agencies that exercised control over colonized territories supporting such endeavors as voyages to test methods of measuring longitude (1761–64); expeditions to measure the transit of Venus (1761 and 1769); Cook's three exploration voyages (1768–79); and the HMS *Bounty* breadfruit mission to Tahiti (1787–89).[4] But such activities, pursued as matters of state policy, came relatively late to Portugal. Only during the reign of Queen Maria I (1777–1816) did royal authorities express a marked interest in systematically gathering data about flora and fauna from across the empire, considering them in terms other than as mere mercantile commodities.[5] Through their actions, imperial administrators in Portugal during the last quarter of the eighteenth century appear to have developed a new appreciation for the potential of organized collecting of information regarding indigenous medicinal substances from the colonies. If gathered and studied in a comprehensive empirical way, they reasoned, such information might support the Portuguese colonial enterprise, broadly defined, and make it more profitable by keeping personnel, slave and free, healthy and on task.[6]

To understand Azeredo and his achievement, we must place him in the context of these times and the extraordinary scientific ferment that was taking place around him, across western Europe and throughout the Portuguese-speaking world.

Although in northern Europe the tenets of empiricism had become firmly established by the late seventeenth century, in continental Portugal, open, systematic scientific inquiry was made possible only with the institutional reforms initiated by the Marquês de Pombal during the third quarter of the eighteenth century. However, experimentation and innovation had long been easier to pursue in the colonies, owing to a combination of pure pragmatic need and a certain liberating distance from ecclesiastical authorities in the metropole, who exercised control over medical education and the circulation of ideas from outside Roman Catholic Europe.[7] Azeredo's scholarly tendencies were driven in part by his exposure to robust scientific inquiry during his years as an impressionable medical student in Edinburgh (1786–88) and young graduate in Leiden (1788), but he also found great freedom to innovate as a young independent physician in Angola, where he served as the chief medical authority in the colony (1790–97).[8]

Azeredo's work in Brazil and Angola is so compelling because he represents, and is a product of, a watershed moment in Portuguese medical history; his career offers a window into a brief era when medical understanding was in profound transition, on the cusp of methodological breakthroughs made possible not only by improved technologies of measuring minute processes of the human organism, but also by a changing culture that was becoming more open—and permissive of scientific inquiry. Raised in colonial Brazil's relatively cosmopolitan capital, Rio de Janeiro, trained in medicine in Scotland and the Netherlands by some of the most advanced medical theorists of the age,[9] and posted to Angola as a colonial chief physician at the height of the transatlantic slave trade, Azeredo gained by these experiences a unique perspective on Atlantic World colonial medicine—as well as a pivotal place in it. His career is illustrative of how Western medicine was changing, in part through increasingly complex interactions between Europeans and indigenous peoples in a broader, botanically richer global context.

Thus, Azeredo's two publications—to test the salubrious qualities of air in Brazil and describing his treatment of fevers in Angola—can be seen as the culmination of an evolving centralized and strategic Portuguese colonial health policy established in Lisbon through the mandates of the Marquês de Pombal, the monarchy, and the Conselho Ultramarino (the Overseas Council, the Portuguese royal administrative directing body for colonial policy[10]), all of which enjoined colonial medical authorities to gather health care data systematically and disseminate their findings for the benefit of the entire imperial enterprise.

Sustained high losses of human capital in the tropical colonies—not only among European soldiers, administrators, and settlers, but also among valuable enslaved persons shipped as merchandise across the At-

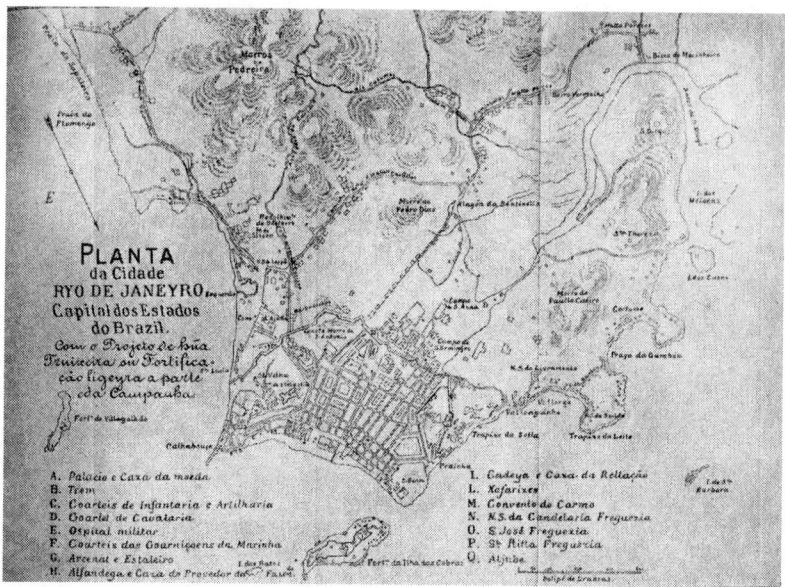

Map of Rio de Janeiro, by Sargento-Môr Francisco José Roscio,
military engineer. "Plan of the City of Rio de Janeiro Capital of the States
of Brazil. With a Project for a Trench." Ink on parchment, 1769.
(Mapoteca do Itamaraty, Rio de Janeiro; public domain
through Wikimedia Commons.)

lantic and Indian Oceans—prompted this initiative. Typically during
the sixteenth to eighteenth centuries, new European and enslaved African arrivals to the Portuguese colonies suffered shockingly high rates
of mortality, their ranks shrinking rapidly owing to traumatic acclima-
tization, brutal working conditions, and tropical diseases.[11] According
to one contemporary estimate, in the three decades between 1604 and
1634, Portuguese military deaths in India exceeded twenty-five thousand men in the Royal Military Hospital of Goa alone.[12] Eventually
the Conselho Ultramarino, desperate to find effective remedies that
could reduce casualties, commissioned medical authorities in Brazil and
Goa to write descriptions of all the medicinal native plants and roots
in their respective areas.[13] Azeredo's work expanded the geographic
coverage of this effort by addressing medical resources and practices in
coastal West Africa.

Other Lusophone physicians and surgeons, notably in Brazil, had compiled similar material for publication, sometimes decades before Azeredo's birth. Azeredo stands out because he went well beyond describing useful medicinal herbs and simples. By contrast, he detailed not only his innovative medical techniques (undertaken in response to the unique health care imperatives he confronted as a result of the physical and social circumstances of colonial Luanda), but the scholarly rationale and apparatus behind them. Further, Azeredo supported his commentary with references to internationally known medical authorities whose works he had encountered in the lecture halls of Edinburgh and Leiden. Among contemporary Portuguese colonial medical practitioners, his cosmopolitan influences and engagement were highly unusual.

Azeredo's ideas and techniques developed through practical direct treatment of untold thousands of patients in Angola: principally Africans, but also European colonists.[14] With the weight of his experience behind him, Azeredo assessed and challenged the contemporary experts' theories, ridiculing some and praising others in the process of defending his own medical methods.

To better understand how the Portuguese imperial strategy in pursuit of improved health and science worked on a global scale, we may consider the activities of some of Azeredo's predecessors and contemporaries in other parts of the Lusophone world. Their efforts provide a telling comparison. How did they respond to Crown requests for medical information from around this vast, diverse maritime empire?

One factor we must bear in mind is that a simple lack of trained European medical practitioners hastened the adoption of indigenous medicines; few doctors and surgeons could be induced to leave the relative comforts of continental Portugal for service in the colonies. Even the most economically dynamic area of the Portuguese colonial system during the eighteenth century, Brazil, had difficulty in attracting licensed physicians and surgeons. In 1783, Belém do Pará had two physicians, seven surgeons, and six pharmacists for a population of eleven thousand; in 1789, four physicians served in the new colonial capital, Rio de Janeiro, but that number increased to nine by 1794. Recife never had more than three or four licensed practitioners at one time during the entire eighteenth century.[15] Those few Portuguese medical practitioners who did take up residence in Brazil during the 1700s continued to gather knowledge about South American materia medica. Some produced handbooks, papers, or guides about the novel indigenous healing plants they encountered.[16] A few with a scholarly bent went much further, creating detailed works for publication, in the hope of achieving a wide audience among interested "botanizing" researchers back in Europe. Azeredo is product of this era and culture.

In 1735, Portuguese-born surgeon Luís Gomes Ferreira brought out his magnum opus, *Erário mineral* (Mineral treasury), an ambitious, eclectic work published in Lisbon.[17] This rare book is one of the first practical comprehensive treatises in the Portuguese language describing Brazilian medical techniques. Ferreira trained as a barber-surgeon at the royal Todos os Santos hospital in Lisbon before settling in 1710 in Minas Gerais, the mountainous mining region northwest of Rio de Janeiro, where he worked as a surgeon for nearly two decades. *Erário mineral* relates Ferreira's long medical experience with the region's diverse population: European settlers, Amerindians, and Afro-Brazilian slaves. Ferreira provided a detailed description of the principal illnesses endemic to colonial southeast Brazil, and also described the most effective regional curing techniques and remedies, often drawn from the blended healing traditions of his disparate patients.[18] Ferreira includes a broad inventory of local medicines and healing compounds, together with explanations of their effects and applications. *Erário mineral* describes the incredibly difficult frontier mining conditions under which slaves worked; this, Ferreira noted, contributed to their chronic ailments. Such conditions prompted European colonists to incorporate various native healing plants into their own medical practices.[19] This incisive treatise thus blends European scientific knowledge with popular medicine from across colonial Brazil's social spectrum.

Of the many expeditions through the Brazilian interior during the colonial period, only a few were initiated as a matter of explicit state policy.[20] The nine-year "philosophical journey" of Dr. Alexandre Rodrigues Ferreira stands out for this reason. For his exceptional medical and botanical discoveries, Brazilians today remember Ferreira as their first great native-born naturalist. Born in 1756 in Salvador da Bahia and sent to Portugal to complete his studies, Ferreira attained the degree of doctor in natural history from the University of Coimbra in 1779. Subsequently he was employed at the royal botanical gardens of the Ajuda Palace in Lisbon, where he gained favor with Queen Maria I, who in 1778 had founded the Royal Academy of Sciences in Lisbon.[21] In 1783, Dona Maria selected Ferreira to lead an expedition to map the barely known Brazilian interior, searching for natural resources that could be profitably exploited. Ferreira's odyssey would traverse the territories of Grão-Pará, Rio Negro, Mato Grosso, and Cuiabá. His traveling apothecary chest included medicines from all over the Portuguese empire, but he soon came to experiment with many native plants that he encountered along the way.[22] Ferreira's expedition reports circulated widely in the Lusophone Atlantic world, thus spreading information about the remedies he had found and tested.[23]

In 1788, Brazilian physician and natural scientist Bento Bandeira de Mello, responding to an explicit royal order, submitted a lengthy memorandum to the Conselho Ultramarino on frequently used indigenous medicines in the coastal northeast of Brazil. He had been charged with creating an alphabetical list of medicinal plants, fruits, and roots from the territories of Pernambuco and Paraíba, with comments about their curative effects.[24] His annotated roster contains fifty-nine different South American healing plants. De Mello sent specimens of many of these plants to the Ajuda Palace royal botanical garden in Lisbon, where they were assessed for their medical usefulness and suitability for transplant to other imperial regions.[25] The desired strategic end of de Mello's efforts, of course, from the perspective of the Conselho Ultramarino, was to further Portuguese aims by reducing chronic wastage of human resources through wounds, injury, and illness.

Another ambitious project of pharmacological botany, *History of the Vegetable, Animal and Mineral Kingdoms, Pertaining to Medicine*, was undertaken by Francisco Arsenio de Sampaio, a Portuguese-born physician who held the post of surgeon at the Hospital of São João de Deus in Cachoeira, the main agricultural market town in the Bahian hinterland, for nearly two decades in the late eighteenth century.[26] Sampaio compiled this multivolume work between 1782 and 1789. Because of its structure and scope, the project appears to have been produced under commission, at the behest of colonial authorities in Bahia or Lisbon. Two extant tomes, handwritten and bound together with stunning original painted illustrations of Brazil's flora and fauna, each contain highly detailed descriptions of a variety of native plants, a summary of their healing virtues, proper doses to administer to patients, and application methods for each remedy.[27] This painstakingly composed work seems to have been intended for publication, aimed at a broad readership in the transatlantic scientific community. The plants described in Sampaio's first volume are organized into twelve sections according to their contemporary medicinal applications. For example, astringent, anti-venom, anti-colic, antispasmodic, purgative and anti-venereal plants are each treated in their own discrete chapters.[28] Unfortunately, Sampaio's labor was not published until the late twentieth century; it remains virtually unknown outside of Portuguese-language scholarship.[29]

In 1785, another Portuguese-born *médico* who had served in Brazil, Manuel Joaquim Henriques de Paiva, published *Farmacopéa lisbonense*, a compendium of medicinal plants and remedies found throughout the Lusophone world.[30] This work drew heavily on Paiva's experience in South America. The author, another of Azeredo's notable medical contemporaries, explained the healing properties of dozens of traditional Brazilian remedies and individual plant drugs in exceptional detail, assessing their utility and prescribing effective methods of application.[31] Paiva benefited from his privileged position as *médico da câmara* (personal physician) of the prince regent, Dom João VI, and he would accompany the Portuguese royal family when they relocated the court to Rio de Janeiro in 1808. *Farmacopéa lisbonense*, based on firsthand experiences and observation, exemplified an empirical approach to the adaptation of indigenous medicine. This guide was widely distributed in Portugal and Brazil; more than any other published work of the eighteenth century, it provided accurate medical information about drugs from Portuguese South America.[32]

During the closing years of the eighteenth century, the diplomat and statesman Dom Rodrigo de Sousa Coutinho (1755–1812), one of the principal advisers to Queen Maria I and the prince regent, Dom João, would become a key advocate for Crown support of scientific inquiry in the Portuguese colonies. He saw clearly the utility of conducting medical surveys across the empire in search of healing commodities that could be used to achieve imperial goals.[33] As a youth, Sousa Coutinho had spent time in Angola, where his father, Francisco Inocêncio de Sousa Coutinho, was governor from 1764 to 1772. Dom Rodrigo himself became overseas minister from 1796 to 1800, followed by a term as treasury minister from 1800 to 1803.[34] In Lisbon he founded Enlightenment-era organizations like the Casa Literária do Arco do Cego, an innovative publisher of technical and scientific texts (mainly concerning agriculture, biology, and botany in Brazil),[35] and the Sociedade Marítima, Militar e Geográfica, charged with overseeing production of charts and maps for all branches of the Portuguese military.[36] As overseas minister, he would have had a deciding role regarding Azeredo's appointment to Angola, and taken an active interest in his publications and activities in Luanda. Sousa Coutinho's cousin, Dom Luís Pinto de Sousa, state secretary of war and foreign affairs in 1789, was also likely a patron of Azeredo's appointment to Angola.[37]

Just before the turn of the nineteenth century, the newly appointed colonial governor of the Maranhão district, Dom Diogo de Sousa, commissioned several descriptive works regarding Brazilian plants that could serve for commerce or medicine. Agents began to compile this information in the forests of the district in 1798; instructions to promote this project had apparently come directly from the Conselho Ultramarino. Three studies arrived in Lisbon by 1801—two folios of watercolor botanical illustrations and one manuscript describing the plants' uses.[38] The two compilations of plant illustrations, together containing some fifty-five varieties in all, focus mainly on species that had indigenous medical applications. These include the stimulant *guaraná*, a widely used healing shrub called *pau d'arco*, and flora to alleviate fevers, asthma, urinary problems, skin disorders, and even to promote hair growth.[39] Vicente Jorge Dias Cabral, a Coimbra University philosophy graduate turned amateur botanist, compiled the thirty-page manuscript, titled "Botanical Guide to Some Plants from the Interior of Piauí." Cabral's text describes the appearance and application of twenty-three medicinal plants.[40]

Portuguese Crown interest in developing improved tropical health care and seeking useful indigenous medical remedies was not limited to colonial Brazil; during Azeredo's time, the royal effort extended to every part of the empire, and even to territories beyond their sovereign control.[41] Because of continuing problems with the health of soldiers and colonial officials everywhere in the tropics, imperial authorities in Lisbon extended their interest in discovering new indigenous remedies to India and China, as well.[42] In a royal directive dated 2 April 1798, Queen Maria I and the Conselho Ultramarino commissioned the Goa Military Hospital's staff physicians and surgeons to write a description of all the useful medicinal plants found along India's southwest Malabar Coast and in the remaining Portuguese enclaves. The following year, chief surgeon Dr. Francisco Manuel Barroso da Silva and his colleagues produced a report, extending to nearly forty manuscript pages, in which they provided thorough descriptions of eleven important roots and plants then in use in the medical facilities of Goa, Damão, and Diu, as well as the East African colonial holdings.[43] The text names these plants as *raiz de cobra* (snake root); *calumba*; *butua* (also known as *pereira brava*); *João Lopes pinheiro*; *pedra quadrada*; *casca de raiz de inhaca*; *bangue*; *cuia cuia*; *batatinha*; *contos do espinhos*; and *inhofancos*.[44]

The 1799 Barroso da Silva report expanded and updated a document submitted in 1794 by the then chief physician of the Portuguese Empire in Asia (the *Estado da Índia*), Ignácio Caetano Afonso, titled "Descriptions and Virtues of Medicinal Roots."[45] Afonso, a native Goan Christian whose medical training consisted of a mixture of European and indigenous healing techniques,[46] had detailed five medicinal roots found in the Indian Ocean basin that he thought would be of use to Portuguese colonial installations in the tropics. Many of the roots he named were in fact of East African origin but had long been growing in southwest India, brought by trade or deliberate transplantation, and used traditionally as ingredients for folk remedies.[47]

So, in context, José Pinto de Azeredo's activities in Angola and Brazil can be seen as part of a much broader strategic effort to preserve fragile human capital within the Portuguese empire by improving the health conditions and quality of care available—in no small part through a deliberate policy of reliance on indigenous medicinal substances and methods. This program, though somewhat improvised and informal, was nevertheless coordinated centrally from the highest levels of government in the metropole. The Crown and its ministers pursued this program with a comprehensive goal in mind: to improve imperial fortunes by protecting and preserving the health of Portuguese subjects abroad—those souls who made the colonial system function.

Azeredo's medical training may also be considered in a broader context. He and his brother were among a significant group of Portuguese subjects to travel to northern Europe for medical studies in the eighteenth century. In fact, Azeredo followed a well-worn path; Portuguese medicine benefited greatly from expatriate physicians and surgeons, many of them *conversos* fleeing Inquisition persecution, who chose to study in the less intellectually restricted environment of Protestant Europe.[48] During the 1700s, London became an important destination for Portuguese New Christians who emigrated out of fear of arrest by the Holy Office. There, along with coreligionists from Spain and Italy, these religious refugees were able to practice Judaism openly and build a tightly knit community within London's cosmopolitan, relatively tolerant environment.[49] In the process, they became foreign-influenced *estrangeirados*, who would in turn serve as conduits bearing innovative healing ideas and methods through correspondence with their colleagues in Roman Catholic Iberia.[50]

Jacob de Castro Sarmento, for example, was one of the most influential Portuguese thinkers to facilitate the flow of medical information into Portugal from northern Europe during the eighteenth century. He spent over forty years in England, from 1721 until 1762, but maintained strong links with a group of progressive-thinking Portuguese intellectuals at home: doctors, officials, and aristocrats who advocated more open policies toward learning and medical practices.[51] In 1725, the Royal College of Physicians in London approved Castro Sarmento as a member, allowing him to practice medicine throughout Britain. Five years later, in recognition of his experimental work with new drugs and treatments, he was elected a fellow of London's Royal Society. Marischal College of the University of Aberdeen granted Castro Sarmento a doctoral degree in 1739.[52]

Prominent among Castro Sarmento's colleagues were numerous Portuguese expatriate medical practitioners, such as David de Chaves and Fernando Mendes. Most notably, there was the brilliant António Nunes

Ribeiro Sanches, who came to London in 1726 before furthering his medical studies in Paris and Leiden; he went on to become a physician of the Imperial Russian court. From Saint Petersburg and later Paris, Ribeiro Sanches would wield a powerful influence on the movement for Portuguese medical reform as well, writing several published treatises advocating improved medical education and public health measures.[53] Ribeiro Sanches's uncle, the *médico* Samuel Nunes Ribeiro, also lived in London, as did his cousin, Isaac de Sequeira Samuda, another active and noteworthy medical researcher.[54]

Azeredo's work may be fitted into the developing intellectual context of the Enlightenment-era Portuguese Atlantic World in other ways. His book on fevers raised awareness about methods to treat and contain contagious disease in Portugal, especially those arriving with transient travelers. Such awareness in turn was part of the motivation for creating a dedicated maritime quarantine station near Lisbon in 1814 at Porto Brandão on the southern banks of the Tagus River, for interning sick passengers aboard ships arriving from the colonies or other countries.[55] Treatment of patients' fevers at Porto Brandão owed no small part to methodologies that Azeredo pioneered and disseminated through his 1799 publication.

As a final point, I must note the key significance of Azeredo's posting to Luanda, a pivotal node in the transatlantic slave trade during the closing decade of the eighteenth century. As a source of enslaved laborers, Luanda held a central, indispensable position in the seaborne colonial system and commercial networks of the Portuguese Atlantic. During Azeredo's tenure, this port served as the primary departure point for slave labor to the plantations and mines of Brazil, as well as other Atlantic colonies controlled by the Dutch, French, and British.[56] The Portuguese colonial economy in the Atlantic was built upon, and could not have functioned without, enslaved labor from Africa—which by the mid-1700s came principally from Angola. A popular contemporary proverb in Brazil went: "Without sugar, no Brazil; without slaves, no sugar; without Angola, no slaves."[57] Slave exports from Luanda averaged well over twenty thousand persons annually during Azeredo's time there, which coincided with the very peak of the transatlantic slave trade.[58]

Thus, the young doctor had ample opportunity to learn about and treat a broad range of disease conditions among captive peoples who had been force-marched from the Angolan interior to the Luanda waterfront holding pens (*feitorias*). Part of his duties, after all, was to ensure the slaves' health so that human merchandise could be taken aboard ship without fear of fever spreading through the valuable cargo. Luanda therefore afforded Azeredo with constant exposure to the diverse healing cosmologies of indigenous Angolans.[59] He noted with frustration how many European colonists, tempted by native curing methods, often turned to them when sick, and suffered as a result.[60]

Significantly, in his practice Azeredo himself, like his predecessors, for the most part eschewed the numerous types of medicinal plants employed by indigenous peoples in Angola. The majority of drugs he used came from South America (quinine) or India (opium), thus exemplifying the interconnected nature of medicinal commerce within the contemporary Portuguese world. Internal evidence from *Maladies of Angola* seems to indicate that Azeredo applied few distinctly indigenous African medicinal substances when treating his patients; he refers to only a handful that he accords therapeutic value.[61] Unlike Portuguese enclaves in India, China, or Brazil, those in West Africa did not export much in the way of natural medical commodities—at least not those meant for use by European practitioners.[62]

When considered alongside the large military hospitals or Jesuit and Santa Casa de Misericórdia installations in Goa, Macau, Salvador de Bahia, and Rio de Janeiro,[63] the medical facilities where Azeredo practiced at Luanda were modestly sized and equipped by comparison. Conditions and resources in Angola simply could not match those of colonial enclaves with larger communities of Portuguese settlers. Additionally, ship arrivals directly from Europe were relatively rare events in Angola by the late eighteenth century; most trading vessels were slave ships from Brazil, while those from the metropole had usually visited Brazil first. Counterclockwise wind and current patterns in the South Atlantic dictated that sailing vessels from Europe would normally travel first to South America before attempting a passage to Angola.[64] Consequently, Azeredo could expect few medical supplies and no fresh medicines from Lisbon. However, this circumstance supported

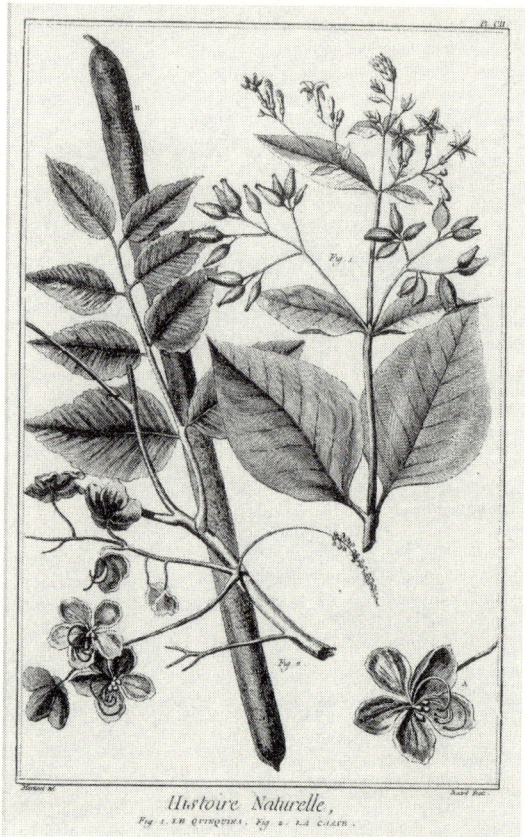

Illustrations of cinchona (fig. 1, *right*) and cassia (fig. 2, *left*).
Engraving originally published in "Histoire naturelle—Règne
végétal," in *Encyclopédie ou dictionnaire raisonné des sciences, des arts
et des métiers*, vol. 6 (plates) (Paris, 1768), plate 102. The Encyclopedia
of Diderot and d'Alembert Collaborative Translation Project
(Ann Arbor: MPublishing, University of Michigan Library, 2010).

his heavy reliance on medicines from Brazil, most notably quinine-
containing cinchona bark and *jalapa*.[65]

José Pinto de Azeredo came of age professionally when the Atlantic World was becoming smaller and increasingly interconnected. His
publications addressed practical problems in health care and science
with methods that he could reasonably hope might be replicated and

applied in Portuguese sovereign territories scattered across four continents. Moreover, in publishing his works when he did, Azeredo could have enjoyed the realistic expectation that he might influence thinkers and policy not only within the Lusophone world, but in a wider audience beyond it, as his readership, he knew, could well have included the broad European learned community with which he had interacted as a medical student.

Azeredo's "Chemical Examination of the Atmosphere of Rio de Janeiro" and *Essays on some Maladies of Angola* represent keystone components of a developing scientific consciousness among elites of the Portuguese empire at the close of the eighteenth century. For Portugal's ruling class and contemporary proponents of a modernized, rationalist approach to imperial development, Azeredo's contributions in science and medicine served as examples of a forward-thinking policy model — a vision long since embraced and well advanced in contemporary Britain, France, and the Netherlands. Moving into the nineteenth century, the competitive commercial success of the Portuguese imperial enterprise would depend on an ability to change and adopt new technologies and even epistemologies — approaches to how knowledge is gathered and used. Azeredo's importance lies in his having helped to set a new tone for Portuguese medicine and science, expediting the transition to a modern empirical era.

Notes

1. Timothy Walker, "Acquisition and Circulation of Medical Knowledge within the Portuguese Colonial Empire during the Early Modern Period," in *Science, Power and the Order of Nature in the Spanish and Portuguese Empires*, ed. Daniela Bleichmar, Kristin Huffine, Paula De Vos, and Kevin Sheehan (Stanford, CA: Stanford University Press, 2009), pp. 247–53.

2. Eric Lars Myrup, "To Rule from Afar: The Overseas Council and the Making of the Brazilian West, 1642–1807" (doctoral dissertation, Yale University Department of History, 2006), pp. 61–73.

3. The Inquisition in Portugal was not abolished until 1821; government censorship of scientific texts continued until the implementation of a new Liberal constitution the following year. José Sebastião Silva Dias, "Portugal e a cultura europeia: Séculos XVI a XVIII," *Biblos* 28 (Coimbra: Universidade de Coimbra, 1952): pp. 292–97.

4. For commentary on this point see the introduction to James Delbourgo and Nicholas Dew, eds., *Science and Empire in the Atlantic World* (New York: Routledge,

2008), pp. 1–16, and the closing essay in that volume by Margaret C. Jacob, "Science, Global Capitalism and the State," pp. 333–44.

5. A. J. R. Russell-Wood, *The Portuguese Empire, 1415–1808: A World on the Move* (Baltimore: Johns Hopkins University Press, 1998), pp. 176–78.

6. Walker (2009), pp. 257–58, 266–68; Timothy Walker, "The Medicines Trade in the Portuguese Atlantic World: Dissemination of Plant Remedies and Healing Knowledge from Brazil, c. 1580–1830," *Social History of Medicine* 26:3 (2013): pp. 414–20.

7. Walker (2009), pp. 248–50.

8. Manuel Serrano Pinto, Marco António Cecchini, Isabel Maria Malaquias, Lycia Maria Moreira-Nordemann, and João Rui Pita, "O medico brasileiro José Pinto de Azeredo (1766?–1810) e o exame químico da atmosfera do Rio de Janeiro," *Manguinhos: História, Ciências, Saúde* (Fundação Oswaldo Cruz, Rio de Janeiro) 12:3 (September–December 2005): pp. 617–26.

9. For example, the physician William Cullen (1710–90), a professor of medicine at Edinburgh and leading figure in the Scottish Enlightenment, had a tremendous influence on Azeredo's training. See E. M. McGirr and W. Stoddart, "Changing Theories in 18th-Century Medicine: The Inheritance and Legacy of William Cullen," *Scottish Medical Journal* 36:1 (February 1991): pp. 23–26; and R. Stott, "William Cullen and Edinburgh Medicine: A Reappraisal," *Society for the Social History of Medicine Bulletin* 38 (June 1986): pp. 7–9.

10. Myrup, pp. 61–73.

11. Until the early nineteenth century, annual mortality rates of 25 percent to 50 percent were common for newly disembarked European soldiers and African slaves in Portuguese colonial enclaves. For transatlantic slave trade mortality rates see David Eltis, *The Rise of African Slavery in the Americas* (Cambridge: Cambridge University Press, 1999), pp. 68, 159, 185–86. In India, the sixteenth-century Dutch traveler John Huyghen van Linschoten observed that, in the Royal Military Hospital of Goa, "every yeare at the least there entered 500 live men, [who] never come forth till they are dead"; see Arthur Coke Burnell and P. A. Tiele, eds., *The Voyage of John Huyghen Van Linschoten to the East Indies. . . .* 2 vols. (London: Hakluyt Society, 1885), vol. 1, p. 237.

12. Alberto C. Germano da Silva Correia, *La Vieille-Goa* (Bastorá, 1931), pp. 274–75; F. P. Mendes da Luz, ed., "Livro das cidades e fortalezas . . . ," *Studia* 6 (1960): f. 8. The author is grateful to Professor Michael N. Pearson for this reference.

13. See Ignácio Caetano Afonso, *Discripçoens e virtudes das raizes medicinaes* [Descriptions and virtues of medicinal roots], manuscript booklet (1794), HAG MR 175, ff. 219–30. See also references to a similar royal directive, dated 2 April 1798, in HAG Monções do Reino 178B (1798–99), ff. 644–45. For Brazil see Bento Bandeira de Mello, manuscript (1788), Arquivo Nacional do Torre do Tombo (ANTT), Ministério do Reino, *caixa* 555, *maço* 444.

14. José Pinto de Azeredo, *Ensaios sobre algumas enfermidades de Angola* (Lisbon: Regia Officina Typografica, 1799), pp. vii–xvi.

15. Conde dos Arcos, memorandum of 8 October 1757, in Eduardo de Castro Almeida, *Inventário dos documentos relativos ao Brasil existantes no Archivo de Marinha e Ultramar de Lisboa*, vol. 1, *Bahia, 1613–1762* (Rio de Janeiro: Officinas Graphicas

da Biblioteca Nacional, 1913), document 2917, pp. 255–56; Licurgo de Castro Santos Filho, *História de medicina no Brazil, do século XVI ao século XIX*, 2 vols. (São Paulo: Editora Brasiliense Ltda., 1947), vol. 1, pp. 50–51.

16. See unpublished manuscripts in the BNRJ: I–47, 19, 20: "*Anotações sobre medicina popular*" (ff. 1–32); and BNRJ: I–47, 23, 5: "*Botânica médica vulgar brasileira: Drogas orgânicas & medicina popular*" (ff. 1–17).

17. Luís Gomes Ferreira, *Erário mineral* (Lisbon: Officina de Miguel Rodrigues, 1735). The Portuguese Crown permitted no printing press in Brazil until 1808, when the royal court took up temporary residence in Rio de Janeiro. Until then, all Brazilian printing projects had to be sent to Lisbon for government approval and typesetting. Thomas E. Skidmore, *Brazil: Five Centuries of Change* (New York: Oxford University Press, 1999), pp. 32–40.

18. See Júnia Ferreira Furtado, "Arte e segredo: O licenciado Luís Gomes Ferreira e seu caleidoscópio de imagens," in *Erário mineral*, 2 vols., coordinated by Júnia Ferreira Furtado (Rio de Janeiro: Editora Fundação Oswaldo Cruz, 2002 [co-edition with the Fundação João Pinheiro and the Fundação de Amparo à Pesquisa of the State of Minas Gerais], vol. 1, pp. 3–30.

19. For examples see Luís Gomes Ferreira, *Erário mineral* (2002), vol. 1, *Tratado III*, pp. 319–446.

20. Such expeditions were usually accomplished by gold- and slave-seeking quasi-military bands of frontiersmen called *bandeirantes*. See Joseph Smith, *A History of Brazil, 1500–2000* (London: Longman, 2002), pp. 10–12, 16–17.

21. Nisia Trindade Lima, director, *A ciência dos viajantes: Natureza, populaces, e saúde em 500 anos de interpretações do Brasil* (Rio de Janeiro: Fundação Oswaldo Cruz, 2000), pp. 40–41.

22. Ibid.

23. A full description of his trip, *Diário da viagem filosófica* (Diary of a philosophical journey), was only published in 1887 in the journal of the Instituto Histórico e Geográfico Brasileiro. Hundreds of extraordinary documents from this journey (maps, diaries, and botanical descriptions) are preserved in Brazil's National Library in Rio de Janeiro: BNRJ, Manuscripts Division, Coleção Alexandre Rodrigues Ferreira.

24. Bento Bandeira de Mello, manuscript (1788), ANTT, Ministério do Reino, *caixa* 555, *maço* 444, 24 folios.

25. Ibid., f. 2.

26. BNRJ, MSS I–12,01,019, Francisco Arsenio de Sampaio, *História dos reinos vegetal, animal e mineral* (manuscript compiled at Cachoeira, Bahia, Brazil, 1782 [vol. 1] and 1789 [vol. 2]), vol. 1, pp. 1, 117–24.

27. Ibid.; volume 1 describes medicinal plants in 219 manuscript pages, supported by another 20 pages of color miniature paintings of many of the plants described in the text. Sampaio included an alphabetical index of each plant name (noting their indigenous Tupí and Guaraní names as well) and commented on nonnative medicinal plants (coffee, pepper, and cinnamon) that the Portuguese had introduced from their overseas territories.

28. Ibid., vol. 1, f. 1.

29. Both volumes of Francisco Arsenio de Sampaio's *História dos reinos vegital, animal e mineral, pertencente à medicina* were published together as a special issue of the journal *Anais da Biblioteca Nacional*, vol. 89 (Rio de Janeiro, 1969).

30. Manoel Joaquim Henriques de Paiva, *Farmacopéa lisbonense, ou collecçao dos simplices, preparaçoes e composiçoes mais efficazes e de major uso* (Lisbon: Filippe da Silva e Azevedo, 1785), frontispiece. The full title in English is "Lisbon pharmacopeia, or collection of the most effective and useful simples, preparations, and compositions."

31. Ibid.

32. In 1802 the original printer reissued the work in an expanded, 287-page edition that included corrections of errors in the earlier text: Manoel Joaquim Henriques de Paiva, *Farmacopéa lisbonense, ou collecçao dos simplices, preparaçoes e composiçoes mais efficazes e de major uso* (Lisbon: Filippe da Silva e Azevedo, 1802).

33. Dom Rodrigo de Sousa Coutinho, "Memória sobre o melhoramento dos domínios de Sua Majestade na América," 1797, in *Textos políticos, económicos e financeiros, 1783–1811*, ed. Andrée-Mansuy Diniz da Silva (Lisbon: Banco de Portugal, 1993), tome 2, pp. 7–12, 38–65, 70–76, 89–92, 401–4.

34. The full titles in Portuguese are, respectively, *secretário de estado dos negócios ultramarinos e da marinha* and *secretário da fazenda*.

35. Ana Paula Tudela, Fernanda Maria Guedes de Campos, and Diogo Ramada Curto, *A Casa Literária do Arco do Cego: Bicentenário (1799–1801)* (Lisbon: Imprensa Nacional-Casa da Moeda e Biblioteca Nacional, 1999).

36. Manuel Amaral, "D. Rodrigo de Sousa Coutinho e o exército: As tentativas de reforma do exército, no interior de um projecto global de reformas da sociedade portuguesa de finais do Antigo Regime," in *A Guerra Peninsular, perspectivas multidisciplinares*, 2 vols. (Lisbon: Comissão Portuguesa de História Militar e Centro de Estudos Anglo-Portugueses, 2008) vol. 2, pp. 355–74.

37. Azeredo's manuscript treatise, *Tratado anatómico dos ossos, vasos lymphaticos e glândulas*, most likely composed in Luanda between 1791 and 1797, is dedicated to Dom Luís Pinto de Sousa Coutinho, who at the time was a minister in the royal council of Queen Maria I (the *secretário dos negócios estrangeiros e da guerra*). See *Tratado anatómico. . . .* (manuscript, Lisbon, 1791), Biblioteca Nacional de Portugal [BNP], *códice* 8485//2, ff. 77–87. I am grateful to Dr. Júlio Rodrigues da Costa of the Biblioteca Pública Municipal do Porto for this reference.

38. José E. Mendes Ferrão et. al., *Plantas do Brasil: Flora económica do Brasil no século XVIII; plantas do Maranhão-Piauí* (Lisbon: Chaves Ferreira Publicações, 2002), pp. 9–11.

39. File of twenty-four watercolor illustrations, held in the Arquivo Histórico Ultramarino (AHU-ACL-CU-016, *caixa* 25, D.1311). A contemporary portfolio of thirty-one botanical illustrations from Brazil, called "Plantas do Piauhi," is held at the Library of the Museum of the Royal Botanical Garden, Lisbon (BMJB, Nr. E 166/24).

40. In Portuguese, "Ensaio botanico de algumas plantas de parte interior do Piauí. . . . " by Vicente Jorge Dias Cabral (1801); manuscript also in the AHU under the same collection (AHU-ACL-CU-016, *caixa* 25, D.1311).

41. See William J. Simon, *Scientific Expeditions in the Portuguese Overseas Territories (1783–1808)* (Lisbon: IICT, 1983), pp. 105–30.

42. A series of official letters and directives between Queen Maria I, her ministers, and colonial officials bemoaning the chronic problem of high mortality among European colonists and discussing ways to address it can be found in the *Livros dos monções do reino*, annual volumes of official state correspondence to and from the Estado da Índia, now preserved in the Historical Archive of Goa. For examples, see HAG MR 169A, ff. 308–9 (12 February 1788); HAG MR 173, f. 157 (31 March 1792); HAG MR 177A, f. 212 (14 February 1797); HAG MR 178A, f. 65 (12 July 1797); and HAG MR 179B, ff. 506v.–508v. (16 March 1799).

43. HAG MR 178B (1798–99), ff. 644–64.

44. Ibid.; the cover letter is dated 29 April 1799.

45. HAG MR 175, ff. 220r.–221v.

46. HAG MR 178A, f. 272; letter to the Portuguese secretary of state in Lisbon, Dom Rodrigo de Sousa Coutinho, from the governor of the Estado da Índia, dated 28 April 1799.

47. Timothy Walker, "Supplying Simples for the Royal Hospital: An Indo-Portuguese Medicinal Garden in Goa (1550–1830)," in *The Making of the Luso-Asian World: Intricacies of Engagement*, ed. Laura Jarnagin (Singapore: Institute for Southeast Asian Studies, 2011), pp. 38–40.

48. Maria Benedita Araújo, "Médicos e seus familiares na Inquisição de Évora," in *Comunicações apresentadas ao 1º Congresso Luso-Brasileiro sobre Inquisição*, 3 vols. (Lisbon: Sociedade Portuguesa de Estudos de Século XVIII e Universitária Editora, 1990), vol. 1, pp. 49–72. For examples of *converso* physicians driven into exile by the Inquisition in the eighteenth century see the following cases: Arquivo Nacional do Torre do Tombo (ANTT), Inquisição de Évora, *processo* nos. 5129, 6426, 9728, 3553, and 8686; Inquisição de Coimbra, *processo* nos. 6355, 6057, 7480, 163, 10098, 6312, and 7681; Inquisição de Lisboa, *processo* nos. 9980, 10429, 575, 8013, 9999, 6291, 2456, 3800, 629, 5278, 10073, 515, 6054, 9776, 6375, 3689, 138, 3686, 7178, and 1912.

49. Edgar Samuel, *The Portuguese Community in London (1656–1830)* (London: Jewish Museum of London, 1992), pp. 2–12.

50. Timothy Walker, *Doctors, Folk Medicine and the Inquisition: The Repression of Magical Healing in Portugal during the Enlightenment* (Leiden: Brill Academic Publishers, 2005), pp. 52–54, 118–46.

51. Richard Barnett, "Dr. Jacob de Castro Sarmento and Sephardim in Medical Practice in 18th-Century London," *Transactions of the Jewish Society of London* 27 (1982): pp. 84–87; Samuel, pp. 84–114.

52. This he earned by correspondence upon the payment of a fee and the submission of evidence of his intense scientific research. Castro Sarmento was thus the first Jew in the United Kingdom to attain such an elevated academic degree. The famous Dr. Samuel Johnson held a low opinion of this practice of effectively selling academic credentials and quipped that some Scottish universities "grew wealthy by degrees." See Samuel, pp. 10–11.

53. António Nunes Ribeiro Sanches, *Tratado do conservação da Saude dos Povos*. . . . (Paris, 1756); *Cartas sobre a educação da mocidade*. . . . (Paris, 1759); *Método para aprender e estudar a medicina* (Paris, 1763).

54. Barnett, p. 84.

55. *Porto Brandão, A Terra e o Tejo* (Almada: Centro de Arqueologia de Almada, 2007), pp. 5–7, 11–12.

56. Herbert S. Klein, *The Atlantic Slave Trade* (Cambridge: Cambridge University Press, 1999), pp. 196–97; David Eltis, *The Rise of African Slavery in the Americas* (Cambridge: Cambridge University Press, 2000), p. 257.

57. In Portuguese: "Sem açucar, não tem Brasil; sem escravos, não tem açucar; sem Angola, não tem escravos." See Stuart Schwartz, "Brazil," in *A Historical Guide to World Slavery*, ed. Seymour Drescher and Stan Engerman (New York: Oxford University Press, 1998), pp. 100–102.

58. David Eltis, Stephen D. Behrendt, David Richardson, and Herbert S. Klein, eds., *The Trans-Atlantic Slave Trade Database* (Open Source Database, www.slave voyages.org); Klein, pp. 196–97.

59. From a wide literature on this subject, an idea of what Azeredo experienced can be gleaned from Kalle Kananoja, "Healers, Idolaters, and Good Christians: A Case Study of Creolization and Popular Religion in Mid-Eighteenth Century Angola," *International Journal of African Historical Studies* 43:3 (2010): pp. 443–65; James H. Sweet, *Domingos Alvares, African Healing, and the Intellectual History of the Atlantic World* (Chapel Hill: University of North Carolina Press, 2011), pp. 111–45; and Luis Nicolau Parés and Roger Sansi, eds., *Sorcery in the Black Atlantic* (Chicago: University of Chicago Press, 2011), chapters 1, 3 and 4.

60. Azeredo (1799), pp. 52–54.

61. For example, Azeredo mentions explicitly the medicinal bark of the *cassoneira* tree in company with other useful trees in a brief passage; Azeredo (1799), pp. 42–45.

62. Walker (2009), pp. 260–65.

63. Figures for the annual number of patients treated at the military hospital in Goa at the end of the eighteenth century, for example, reveal that this was a very high-capacity institution; see HAG MR 173, f. 168 (3,476 patients in 1791); HAG MR 176B, f. 436 (3,858 patients in 1793); HAG MR 176B, f. 448 (3,076 patients in 1794); and HAG MR 177A, f. 218 (1,932 patients in 1797). Contemporary figures for hospitals in Salvador, Rio de Janeiro, and Macau would be proportionate but comparable.

64. Russell-Wood, pp. 31–39; Dava Sobel and William J. H. Andrewes, *The Illustrated Longitude* (New York: Walker and Co., 1998), pp. 8–9.

65. See Walker (2013), pp. 428–30.

Describing and Explaining

The Systematic Horizon of the *Essays* by José Pinto de Azeredo

Adelino Cardoso

(Centro de História d'Aquém e d'Além-Mar & Faculdade de Ciências Sociais e Humanas), Universidade Nova de Lisboa

It is not enough for us to have knowledge of palpable things;
our senses are few and imperfect and are of little use unless
they are guided by reason, which is more sublime.
—José Pinto de Azeredo, *Essays on Some Maladies of Angola*

José Pinto de Azeredo, Teacher and Observer

E ssays on Some Maladies of Angola is the result of a diligent and methodical effort by a qualified doctor who was educated in the best schools of his day, and in which he limits himself to the narration of facts and the analysis of phenomena with the pragmatic intuition to uncover the best therapies for the illnesses in question.[1] Much of this work's value rests precisely here: in the accuracy of his observations and clinical investigation. However, despite declaring that "the work I present to you is only my observations" (p. 64), *Essays* is much more than a mere pragmatic-descriptive record; it offers us a much broader vision of the medical arts and sciences. Azeredo assumes the role of both observer and teacher, and also that of physiologist: he is an observer in the sense that, following a plan, he systematically analyzes and records phenomena; a teacher in that, given the extent of his knowledge and the effectiveness of his remedies, he is responsible for training young doctors; and a physiologist because he is a researcher seeking to provide an integrated view of the human body and the mechanisms through which it performs those operations essential to the preservation of life and health.[2]

Azeredo had a view of the contemporary state of medicine that was typical of the Enlightenment. He followed the advance of science and its struggle against obscurantism and preconception.[3] A lucidly critical spirit, Azeredo resisted the temptation of dogma, and recognized that the most advanced state of human knowledge is not constituted in absolute and definitive truths, but rather in taking new steps on the path to progress, which was made possible only through all that had gone before. It is certain that William Cullen, whom Azeredo calls his "wise master" (p. 77), would not be the "creator and father of modern medicine" (p. 80) that Azeredo sought to follow had Herman Boerhaave not already destroyed "all of his predecessors' systems" (p. 79). In effect, the mistakes of the past, as well as those of the time in which Azeredo was writing, fulfilled an indispensable heuristic function in an intrinsically controversial process, as is explicitly stated in connection to one of the book's central theses — the proximate cause of tetanus: "while the idea I propose may be a delusion, it will at least serve to provoke great minds to try to understand the error and to discover the truth" (p. 126).

The most basic condition of scientific discourse is that it be subject to proof, given that the natural imperfection of the human spirit means that such discourse is liable to many errors and, moreover, that preconceptions shaping our ideas often lead to the fogging of observed phenomena.[4] Similarly, medical tradition must be viewed critically, submitting its procedures and doctrines to examination, however deeply rooted they are, even among the more free and open spirits.[5] Consequently, Azeredo's Enlightenment confidence in science and progress is tempered by a keen sense for the limits of human knowledge.

Experience Tempered by Reason: Beyond Mere Experience

The reader of Azeredo's *Essays* cannot but sense the great affinity between them and Kant's *Critique of Pure Reason* (1781). There is a shared ambience between the authors, for whom the difference between empiricists and rationalists is entirely pointless, making it necessary to unite reason with experience instead of concentrating on their duality. Like Kant,[6] Azeredo viewed experience as the starting point for understanding, while also acknowledging that *mere experience* is not enough to produce science.[7]

For Kant, the process of understanding took place through the union of experience and reason, given that, in the language of the German philosopher, "our cognition arises from two fundamental sources"— sensibility and understanding.[8] The contribution of each of these— intuitions and concepts, respectively—is equally indispensable: "Without sensibility no object would be given to us, and without understanding none would be thought. Thoughts without content are empty, intuitions without concepts are blind."[9] Azeredo also established a very close correlation between theory and practice in the constitution of natural science. He employed the discipline of the methodical observer: "Up to now I have not departed from a narration of facts and have sought to avoid all conjecture and speculation. I have merely recounted with care and caution the observations made during my study" (p. 78). Gathering facts is a requirement of scientific labor: the problem, however, is that facts do not explain themselves, and that it is therefore important to look beyond them. Hence, in the next part of the text, Azeredo differentiates between the scientific and the empirical method, demanding an inalienable place for theoretical elaboration.[10] Because it is not possible to separate them from practice, theories are essential to the process of creating science: there is no good practice without theoretical support to organize and make sense of the phenomena. Metaphysics is the researcher's demand to open new horizons and to see beyond the visibility of immediate experience.

Philosophy, understood in the Enlightenment and Kantian manner as a critical-methodological endeavor, rather than the systematic conception of philosophy as a view of the world, has a founding and guiding role in scientific research: "because the philosophizing mind belongs to he who seeks the truth, he who values experience, he who makes discoveries, and he who moves beyond empiricism" (p. 64). The aim of removing that empiricism that only recognizes facts is an invitation to the reader to temper and relativize the reiterated affirmation that the work "contains no more than the result of my experiences" (p. 62); that "I did nothing more than give voice to nature and observe" (p. 64); that "laborious and confident observation is the only way to learn how to seek the methods most suitable for the treatment of the illness" (p. 67). Experience is, effectively, a given, but it is also constructed according to a guiding plan. Hence our medical philosopher's happy synthesis, the purpose of the "only means we have of getting close to [the truth are] . . . experiments, examinations, hypotheses: these are the only means of discovering that which the senses cannot reach" (pp. 125–26). Experiments, examinations, and hypotheses are equally essential for the construction of the scientific edifice.

The distinction between "empiricism" and the "old empirical physicians" (pp. 93–94) quite clearly assumes the form of an attack on the empirical sect in medicine: "where I am unable to discover the truth, I will at least seek to take us away from the old school sect that in centuries past hindered the progress of medicine and of which we should be ashamed to allow to appear in the present" (p. 126). The accusation is very strong: the empirical sect was impeding the progress of medicine, and the existence of writers who defended it in these more enlightened times was cause for shame. This uncompromising position against those physicians whose "treatment . . . far from being established scientifically, is entirely empirical" (p. 126) positions Azeredo close to the "philosophical medicine" promoted by De Bordeu in his *Encyclopédie* article "Crisis," in which he demands a preeminent place for the medical philosopher (in contrast to the simple "popular" physician), who, in his quality as a "great observer," transcends "ordinary limits."[11]

Double Consideration: General and Particular

The coherence of Azeredo's *Essays* rests in the relationship between pathology and therapy. The former is concerned with the study of illnesses, their classification, symptoms, evolution, and, crucially, their causes. Medical good practice is based on the accurate identification of illness and its cause. The four essays into which the book is divided (maladies of Angola, intermittent maladies, dysentery, and tetanus) follow a uniform structure: determination of the cause and the search for effective remedies.

Azeredo begins his examination of the causes of maladies in Angola with a warning relating to the nature of the relationship between cause and effect: "All causes always need the disposition of nature, and because of this they do not always function" (p. 80). In a quite accurate way, Azeredo affirms that the causal relationship is not strictly necessary, since it is subject to contingencies and individual variations. The phrase "disposition of nature" refers precisely to the innate or acquired tendencies of individuals that affect their constitution. Consequently, the explanation for morbific causes implies both an understanding of the illness and the paying of attention to the actual nature of the individual patient.

The examination of the maladies of Angola is more detailed because Azeredo outlines a general framework of the etiology of endemic diseases: that is, those that affect a significant number of individuals and which spread rapidly, such as fevers and dysentery. Azeredo's innovation rests, in this case, in his distancing himself from the humors model that explained morbidity by either an excess or a lack of some of the four humors and which looked for the origins of afflictions in the quality of the air: "I am convinced that endemic illnesses depend on a single common cause that exists in the atmosphere and which is always hidden from us" (p. 81). This general cause is crucial, but ineffective in itself, however: "This general cause will not function without the necessary conditions also existing" (p. 81).

Azeredo goes on to catalog a wide range of determining causes, which he also designates as accidental and exciting, submitting them to debate: "While all the causes mentioned here may or may not be the cause of illness in the country, I dare not address them and leave it to the judgment of the readers to decide" (p. 91). Of these causes, Azeredo mentions contaminated water, excessive heat, the showers that "create a thick and pestilent air that is impossible to breathe" (p. 87), the high number of slaves, the immense amount of putrefying fish, the unburied dead, certain local habits, the plentiful banquets, entire nights without sleep, lack of hygiene, poor diet, and venereal disease. As we can see, the causes listed are of distinct natures: ecological, social, and anthropological.

In relation to the proximate cause of tetanus, Azeredo criticizes the silence of those "writers who have approached this malady" (p. 126), attributing it to the fear they will "enter a chaos of difficulties and problems that are incomprehensible even today" (p. 126). With courage and a sense of risk, Azeredo tries to find a way through highly obscure material. Our philosopher physician effectively followed a procedure that went against the then-dominant humorist school in its most unknown area: the muscles—"the proximate cause of tetanus is the spasmodic contraction of the simple solids [muscles], which lose their flexibility by having received some influences from the vital solids [nerves]" (p. 127). Here Azeredo touches on the most difficult physiology of the second half of the eighteenth century: the connection between the nervous and the muscular systems.

Outline of a Medical System

To crown his *Essays*, in relation to the labyrinthine question of the proximate cause of tetanus, Azeredo ventures into the field of physiology, the flourishing of which gave an important stamp to Enlightenment medicine.[12] The progress of the pathology and of the therapy depends on the progress of the physiology: "The pathology of [muscles] cannot be properly separated from their physiology, and in this respect there has been little progress" (p. 125), Azeredo even states that "we entirely ignore the nature of muscular movements" (p. 125), which is where the challenge facing the developing science of physiology arises, and that may explain the most prodigious natural phenomenon—voluntary movement: "Their prodigious nature in all their functions is never more admirable than in the voluntary movements we give our bodies. We develop theories to explain this phenomenon, but how far from the truth are they?" (p. 125). The difficulty arising from this phenomenon is that it results from the interaction of two great organic systems: the nervous and the muscular, which cannot but be linked in animate bodies "by a cohesive force" (p. 126), which is to say, to complete the integrated totality of the organism.

What then? Everything other than desisting from seeking answers, because to do so would mean keeping human understanding in the "lethargy of the ignorance in which it was born" (p. 126). The path to follow is that of the solidism introduced in the membrane theory developed by Gjuro Baglivi and which was followed by Herman Boerhaave and Albrecht von Haller, among others. In the system sketched out by Azeredo,[13] there is a clear separation in relation to the Hallerian conception of the mutual independence of the muscular and nervous systems, which respond to the primordial functions of irritability and of sensibility. Azeredo was searching for a unitary system—one based on sensibility and which would, therefore, give primacy to it.

From the lexical standpoint, Azeredo called the simple solids "muscles" and the vital solids "nerves": "The solids in our body are divided into the simple and the vital: the former consist of the muscle mass, and the latter constitute a fundamental part of the nerves. 'Simple solids' are found in both animate and inanimate bodies. Nerves are found only in animate bodies" (p. 126). The specific nature of the living body is the result of the nerves and their associated sensibilities. In effect, the nerves are the "sole principle, genesis, and cause of all of our body's actions" (p. 127). The muscles carry out organic actions, for example at the digestive level, an "intervention of the [nerves] with which they are united" (p. 127). Consequently, in his account Azeredo adopts a more typical eighteenth-century physiological approach, one that centers on sensibility.[14]

Conclusion

The fundamental interest of the *Essays* is practical, that is to say, to contribute toward Angola's public health by studying the illnesses that afflict the Angolan people and by searching for the most effective therapies. Without any triumphalism, Azeredo notes the progress that has been made in treating and curing those illnesses with which the book is concerned.[15]

In the Enlightenment fashion, Azeredo demonstrated great confidence in the power of enlightened action. Rather than follow the Hippocratic tradition, which was reinforced by Georg Ernst Stahl, and to which even Cullen was not immune (p. 77), Azeredo played up the role of art over that of nature and stood against the idea that the physician was nature's assistant, and, especially, against the curative power of nature: "This way of explaining nature's actions seems to me to be closest to the truth, and completely undermines the 'healing force of nature' that Cullen, without need, seeks to sustain" (p. 81).

Essays on Some Maladies of Angola is a challenge for the teacher seeking a scientifically grounded therapy, since neither the European medical tradition nor local customs can provide an adjusted understanding: neither bloodletting nor magic has any curative effect.

Azeredo's approach to perfecting the art and science of medicine calls attention to organic, psychosocial, and anthropological factors that imply a conception of medicine as a natural and social science. In fact, health and illness are *complete human phenomena*, which call for an interdisciplinary understanding that reaches beyond the bifurcation between scientific culture and humanistic culture.

Notes

1. "Because my goal is to narrate facts and analyze phenomenon in order to decide the best method of treating diseases, which is the doctor's obligation, what I present here is neither ostentatiously eloquent nor of sublime style" (p. 65).

2. In fact, throughout the eighteenth century and at least until the publication of Claude Bernard's *Leçons de physiologie* (1879), the most common definition of physiology was "the understanding of the laws of life," as can be seen in the preface to the *Dictionnaire des sciences médicales par une societé de médecins et chirurgiens* (Paris: Panckouke, 1814).

3. "It could not be expected that only medicine would remain in its backward state through the continuation of this illuminated and industrious age in which all other arts and sciences are being perfected." (p. 63)

4. "I am sure my discourse contains many lapses and errors and that my conclusions do not always derive from the principles I state. Naturally, the spirit of man is not perfect and is easily inclined to express assumptions" (p. 64).

5. "Some of those writing this century are merely repeating old doctrines rather than reflecting on them, and allow their inviolate respect for their opinions to pass into our days. Even Cullen, my wise master, being a free and eclectic man, fell into the same error concerning the critical days" (p. 77).

6. This is *Critique of Pure Reason*'s starting point: "Experience is without doubt the first product that our understanding brings forth as it works on the raw material

of sensible sensations. . . . Nevertheless, it is far from the only field to which our understanding can be restricted." See Immanuel Kant, *Critique of Pure Reason*, trans. Paul Guyer and Allen Wood (Cambridge: Cambridge University Press, 1998), p. 127.

7. "Physics furnishes us with solid principles from which we take abstract conclusions, and these consequences serve as generic rules that are also new principles in which we discover other physical truths of which our senses are unaware. Thus they are mutually given into our hands and must always remain inseparable. There will never be progress if we use one without the other" (p. 78).

8. Kant, p. 193.

9. Kant, pp. 193–94.

10. "However, seeking to investigate the proximate cause of fevers in order to discover a method of cure that is scientific rather than empirical, I find myself obliged to discourse metaphysically and to draw inferences that serve as generic notions for this same end. Although many argue theories are of no use, I find myself unable to separate them from practice" (p. 78).

11. Théophile De Bordeu, "Crise," in Denis Diderot and Jean Le Rond d'Alembert, *Encyclopédie, ou dictionnaire raisonné des sciences, des arts et des métiers*, vol. 4 (Paris, 1759), p. 405.

12. The reference on this topic is François Duchesneau, *La physiologie des lumières: Empirisme, modèles et théories* (The Hague: Martinus Neuhoff, 1982). For more recent writing see Hubert Steinke, Urs Boschung, and Wolfgang Proß, *Albrecht von Haller: Leben — Werke — Epoche* (Göttingen: Wallstein Verlag, 2008).

13. As noted by Manuel Silvério Marques and António Braz de Oliveira in their study included in this volume, in chapter 2 of "Isagòge pathologica do corpo humano" (1802), Azeredo distinguishes himself from contemporary medical systems in his desire to obtain a conclusive response to organic phenomena. However, while the author rejected the system on the doctrinal level, at the operative level he assumed a systematic procedure, seeking a principle that unified life and its respective functions, placing it on the level of sensibilities, which assumes the status of a primordial function of life.

14. The *Encyclopédie* article on sensibility in its medical sense considers it to be "the base and conservative agent of life, of animality par excellence, the most beautiful and most singular phenomenon." See Henri Fouquet, "Sensibilité, sentiment," in Diderot and d'Alembert, *Encyclopédie*, vol. 15 (Paris, 1765), p. 15.

15. "I was not as successful in the treatment of dysenteries as I was with fevers, despite making the greatest effort possible. . . . I confess my method of treating dysentery is as yet very imperfect. Future experiments and observations will perhaps have more favorable results than those we have experienced until now. . . . In no African illness did I work with so little success for so long as with tetanus, and in no other did I succeed in discovering a treatment as certain" (p. 65).

Shadows in the Enlightenment of Imperial Tropics

José Pinto de Azeredo's *Enfermidades de Angola*

PART I

António Braz de Oliveira

(Biblioteca Nacional de Portugal)

There was much vivacity in [Azeredo's] eyes and expression and
nobility in his face; he was thin and shorter than average; however,
he had a handsome face, was blessed with a jovial nature and with
affable and polished manners. He had a deep and thoughtful spirit,
was passionate and enterprising; he was opinionated and willing
to suffer the greatest privations in order to achieve his goals.[1]

—Emílio Joaquim da Silva Maia, 1840

José Pinto de Azeredo (1764–1810) is not, and never has been, an
illustrious unknown. He is mentioned in public records at the
age of twenty-four, while still a student (1788); he is mentioned a
few months later when he became the physician-general of São
Paulo da Assunção de Luanda (1789); he is mentioned while teaching
rational philosophy and medicine in Angola (1791–97); he is mentioned
when his book, *Essays on Some Maladies of Angola*, was printed (1799); he
was mentioned, finally, when he was appointed physician to the royal
chamber and when the royal family set sail for Brazil (1807), his mother
country, and perhaps where he would have liked to have been buried
three years later.

However, perhaps the first historical tribute to Azeredo's legacy was
delivered a full thirty years after his death, by Emílio Joaquim da Silva
Maia in 1840, in the eulogy quoted above, delivered to the Brazilian

Historical and Geographical Institute and simultaneously published in its *Revista Trimestral*, as well as in the *Revista Médica Fluminense*. It wrongly states that Azeredo was born in 1763, but asserts correctly that he was a contemporary of José de Resende Costa,[2] whom he knew from their days at the school that Silva Alvarenga opened in Rio, and who perhaps was one of those who remembered Azeredo as having "much vivacity in his eyes and expression and nobility in his face," as Silva Maia reported. What is certain is that Silva Maia's "eulogy" became the biographical norm, and through it the chronological mistakes became encyclopedic.[3]

"On the 17th day of May, 1764, I baptized José Inocente . . ."

Today we are able to state that there is reliable testimony that José Pinto de Azeredo was born on 5 May 1764 in the parish of Candelária in Rio de Janeiro.[4] However, the documentary evidence is thus: in the Portuguese national archive there is a copy of his baptism certificate, which his brother Francisco appended to the official *mortis causa* inventory of José Pinto de Azeredo's property.[5] Elsewhere we will attempt to elaborate on this matter, and the rest of what this providentially discovered inventory says regarding Azeredo's life and health.

This document prejudices and perhaps undermines the conjecture that Azeredo was born in 1766.[6] There are also doubts concerning his father's name: Francisco Ferreira de Sousa is what the written record suggests—the "legitimate son of the *graduate* Francisco Ferreira de Sousa . . . and of his wife, Dona Ângela Maria de Morais."[7] The emphasis is justified: we know that the father of José Inocente was said at that time to be the surgeon in the First Regiment of Rio de Janeiro, but we do not know if he was graduated. The same document also states that José Inocente's brother, Francisco, was born four and a half years later, on 4 November 1768.[8]

However, the birth is just the first problem; many doubts remain as we move forward. According to Silva Maia, José de Rezende Costa stated that, through his secondary school studies, Azeredo "demonstrated great aptitude and application, becoming *one of Professor Alvarenga's first* students" [italics added].[9] "One of the first" could mean

32

either one of the first students to attend Alvarenga's school in Rio de Janeiro, or that he was one of the top students in the class in terms of aptitude and application, which is what seems to be the suggestion. As has already been noted,[10] the initial reading raises yet another awkward chronological problem, which is that it is very probable that Silva Alvarenga, coming from Rio das Mortes, arrived in Rio de Janeiro in 1782, and that he began teaching rhetoric that August.[11] By that time Azeredo was eighteen years and three months old. Where had he been before then?

It seems important to find out where and with whom Azeredo attended primary and secondary school, following the tradition of the time.[12] Not being destined for "rustic service," knowing how to read, write, and count (by the age of six or seven, 1770–71) through maternal and paternal devotion, whether or not supplemented with a private tutor, Azeredo, according to Maia, "since his most tender infancy . . . showed a great inclination for education; his father, who loved him very much, threw himself into his education."[13]

Unfortunately, we have no testimonies that suggest the young Azeredo had attended any public secondary school, whether run by the state or by the church, prior to 1782. And if we are able to admit that he learned something about the fabric of the body and the art of curing from his father, then it is also not unreasonable to assume that it was at home that he began to learn the English and French languages that were to prove so useful to him in later years.

After August 1782 he had classes in Latin, moral and rational philosophy, and rhetoric with Silva Alvarenga, as well as other classes with other masters that the common record does not mention. What is certain is that in mid-1786, at the age of twenty-two and seventeen respectively, José and Francisco Pinto de Azeredo[14] traveled to Europe, where they enrolled in Edinburgh University's Faculty of Medicine. Their matriculation records for the years 1786 and 1787 are still held at Edinburgh University.[15]

While in Edinburgh the Azeredo brothers attended lectures on many subjects, particularly anatomy and surgery, chemistry, botany, medicine and pharmacy, medical theory and practice, and clinical medicine, this last at the city's Royal Infirmary.[16] For two entire academic

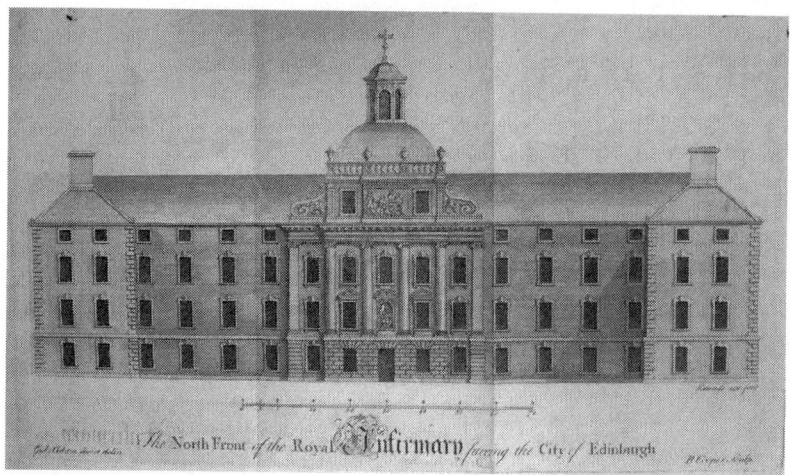

The Royal Infirmary of Edinburgh, Scotland (built 1738), the teaching hospital where José Pinto de Azeredo trained in medicine. Published in William Maitland, *History of Edinburgh from Its Foundation to the Present Time*, 9 vols. (Edinburgh: Hamilton Balfour & Neill, 1753). Monro Collection, Special Collections, Central Library, University of Otago, Dunedin, New Zealand.

years, from October 1786 to May 1788, they were exposed to the lessons of Alexander Monro II, professor of anatomy and surgery; Joseph Black, professor of chemistry; Daniel Rutherford and Francis Home, professors of botany and of materia medica (Home also provided lectures on clinical medicine); William Cullen, professor of the practice of medicine; and James Gregory, professor of the institutes of medicine.[17]

Whether or not they conscientiously attended all the lessons given by these professors, and others that were not part of the obligatory curriculum, is something that we cannot, for now, state with any certainty. However, we read from José Pinto de Azeredo's own hand that, in 1787 or 1788, he attended a lecture in London by John Hunter.[18]

"Upon the whole, all his experiments are conducted with great judgment"

The person who wrote this was Andrew Duncan in the *Medical Commentaries*,[19] referring to José Pinto de Azeredo. If we read correctly the summary Duncan made of Azeredo's paper presented to the Harveian Society of Edinburgh, we can see it was greatly inspired by Joseph Black's "Experiments upon Magnesia Alba, Quicklime, and Some Other Alcaline Substances" (1755).[20] While in Edinburgh, Azeredo produced two other texts, one of which sits well both with those "inferences" Duncan believed "highly important, both in a chemical and medical view" and with our conjecture. We refer to certain *"De Aere* experiments" that Azeredo said were included "in the memoires of the Edinburgh Physics Society for 1788," which are, unfortunately, lost.[21] The other text, now held by the Brazilian Historical and Geographical Archive, is titled *Lexicon nosologicum, morborum definitiones continens, ad medicinae tirones accommodatum*, and had been written in 1787 or 1788, perhaps as an attempt to recollect William Cullen's *Synopsis nosologiae*.[22]

From all these "soul fragments" we now have, for the first time, words, or copies of words, written in José Pinto de Azeredo's own hand. Thus we enter into a biographical history supported by autographic primary sources that are obligatory readings today for a project such as this. If Azeredo was relatively sparing in his references to his own past, in the texts that survive there are, however, moments reflected of his experiences and his journey that are not forgotten and that are not lost to his silence.

What would be significant about Azeredo's time in Edinburgh was his silence about what all his contemporaries had begun to comment on in the meantime (1780–88): Scottish physician John Brown's emerging "Brunonian" system and the particular manner in which the faculty and other critics treated it on that side of the English Channel. In chapter 2 of "Introduction to the Pathology of the Human Body," the written work that best explains his thoughts, Azeredo explains how

Brown's principles are the same as the old [Roman] Methodists.[23] The *strictum* and *laxum* of Themison is Brown's sthenic and asthenic. If Jones is persuaded that these two sects differ greatly between themselves (b) it is because he did not reflect on the fact that Brown was writing in a more enlightened era. . . . Though he speaks of *his extensive practice* where he performed at his maximum, however myself and others who were in Edinburgh at that time know very well that he cured little or nothing.[24]

Very little is known about the Azeredo brothers' lives in Edinburgh, London, or Leiden during the time they were there. We do not know who knew them, how they provided for themselves, where they stayed, how they studied (whether only inside or also outside the universities), to which clubs and societies they belonged,[25] what news they received from Brazil, Portugal, or revolutionary France, and so on.

We do know, however, that they did not complete their course at Edinburgh (which at that time lasted three years) before moving on to Leiden in early June 1788.[26] What is left to us of their time in Leiden is, for now, vague.[27] The diploma was the final step and result of the graduation process that included an academic discussion of Hippocrates's *Aphorisms*. The *historia morborum* (that is, the disease known commonly as gout), about which Azeredo was questioned and on which he was required to speak for an hour, followed the usual order: definition, history, remote cause, proximate cause, and treatment.[28]

"Let it be known . . . that I hereby appoint Dr. José Pinto de Azeredo to the position of physician general of the . . . capital of the Kingdom of Angola"

The course that the young José Pinto de Azeredo followed thereafter leaves no doubt that he was an excellent student when he was at Edinburgh. However, contemporary sources fail to explain his sudden, telling appointment to a demanding royal mission; nor do they confirm that he had gone to study in Edinburgh with royal protection.[29]

What had happened in the meantime? June 1788 was a time of celebration. The brothers had graduated from Leiden, but we do not know whether they returned to Scotland to collect their belongings and to thank their professors and benefactors for their time as students — but we believe that they did. However, if they did, then we do not know to whom, or in what way, exactly, they expressed their gratitude.[30] By January 1789 they were already in Lisbon, and there received a passport allowing them to return to Brazil; on 19 February they received a letter of authorization to practice medicine, signed by the Junta do Protomedicato.[31] On 24 April a royal letter was signed appointing José Pinto de Azeredo to the position of physician general for the Kingdom of Angola. He was not yet twenty-five years old.

However, let us not get ahead of ourselves. Between April 1789 and Azeredo's arrival in Luanda on 27 September 1790, he spent a year and a half in Brazil and published "Chemical Examination of the Atmosphere of Rio de Janeiro" in the *Jornal Enciclopédico*.[32]

We know very little about what Azeredo did during this time in Brazil. Some years later, in his *Essays on Some Maladies of Angola*, he said that "in Rio de Janeiro, in Baía, and in Pernambuco" he had observed the same infirmities that are to be found in Angola, and that he had begun "to put into practice in the city of Rio de Janeiro" the curative method he used, and that the successes he obtained there had convinced him "to continue with their use in Angola."[33]

The next news we have of Azeredo is dated 4 October 1790, when a notice arrived in Lisbon stating that the physician general of Angola had arrived in Luanda on 27 September on the ship *Belém*. However, it was not until 10 September the following year that the governor of Angola instructed that a notice to be read out by criers in towns and villages throughout the land, making it known for all to hear that "His faithful majesty . . . has appointed Dr. José Pinto de Azeredo to the position of physician general in this capital" with "the duty to teach practical medicine with anatomical instruction for the benefit of those who wish to take up the profession."[34]

"Professor of Medicine in the Kingdom of Angola" is how the *Jornal Enciclopédico* described Dr. José Pinto de Azeredo. In the *Oração da sapiêcia* (Prayer for wisdom), Azeredo announced the nature of his program. Following the exhortation to the "dear disciples," it outlined the lesson plan. First anatomy, then physiology, followed by nosology and therapeutics. As expected, in the *Oração* the greatest detail was devoted to anatomy; Azeredo instructed that "the lesson begin with practical medicine and with anatomical instruction."[35] He did not speak here of teaching rational philosophy, nor did it seem reasonable to do so. The reason to mention this, as noted above, came from Azeredo, who, in 1805, stated as much in his application to be appointed physician in Rio

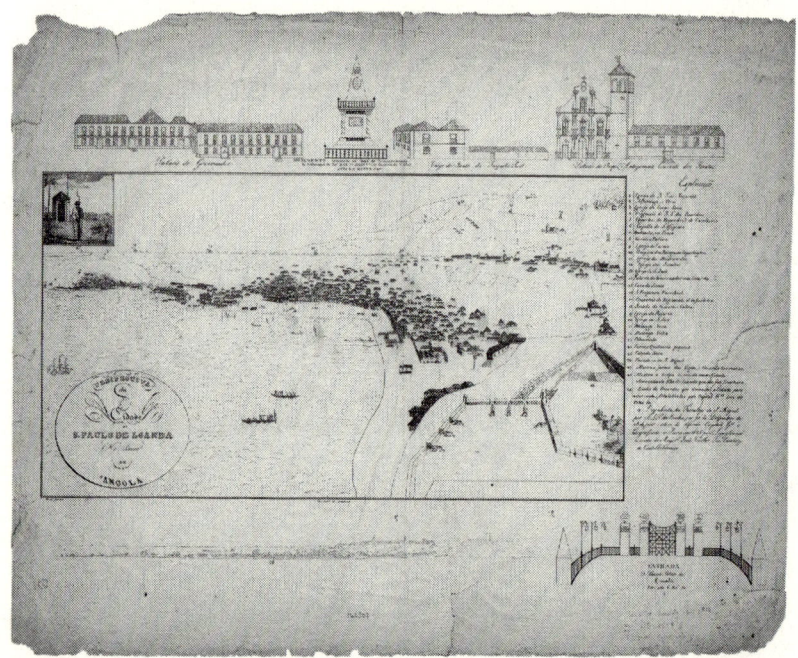

Perspective of the city of São Paulo de Luanda, Angola; elevated and
horizon views, including the Santa Casa da Misericórdia church and hospital
buildings where José Pinto de Azeredo practiced and taught medicine.
Engraving, A. L. P. da Cunha, 1816. Biblioteca Nacional de Portugal:
Ref. Luanda_cc-1698-a_0001_1_p24-c-R0150.

de Janeiro. The physician general was forced to teach the basic elements
of rational philosophy by the condition in which he found education in
the kingdom of Angola.[36]

Azeredo's time in Angola was no holiday. These were the seven most
intense and least healthy years of his life. On his return from Angola
he was ill, perhaps very seriously ill. He kept his suffering to himself.

We do not have enough documents from this period to know how
Azeredo passed his days. If any documents exist that were produced
either by him or for him in the Luanda City Hospital, or in the office
of the colonial government, or in the royal court in Lisbon, they have
yet to be found.

While we have little evidence of how he spent his time, the same is not true of what he wished to leave to posterity. Of the many preparatory writings for his lessons, some that survived elsewhere provide us with detailed information.[37]

However, among all his duties of this time, the highlight must remain the conclusion of *Essays on Some Maladies of Angola*, the only book he published during his life, also with royal patronage. It was brought out by the Royal Typography Office in Lisbon in 1799, two years after his return from Angola.

Below we will look at the contents of this book in more detail. For now it is enough to resume the thread, and to say that we believe that the edition of the *Essays* that was drafted in Luanda must have taken Azeredo around eighteen months to write, from the beginning to the final page (written in Brazil at the end of 1797), to its review by the panel of the General Commission for the Examination and Censorship of Books (mid-1798), to its appearance on the shelves of the bookshops of Lisbon, Oporto, and Coimbra (early 1799).[38]

The illnesses are examined in four essays: on remittent fevers; on intermittent fevers; on dysenteries; and on tetanus. Each of these is subsequently subdivided in line with contemporary academic fashion, as follows: definition; history; proximate cause; remote causes; and cure (in Latin, *definitio*, *historia*, *causa proxima*, *causae remotae*, and *ratio medendi*).

Essays did not go unnoticed. However, for us today it is difficult to assess the immediate reaction to it, particularly among Azeredo's peers. Much that has been written in the medical literature at the turn of the nineteenth century, when not intentionally polemical, chose a disheartening and dilettantish silence toward the work. However, we are certain the book was gratifying to the author. So much so that Azeredo seemed enthused with the work and sought to continue, launching into the editing of "Introduction to the Pathology of the Human Body" (Isagòge patológica do corpo humano) and the "Collection of Clinical Observations" (Coleção de observações clínicas), both prepared to go to press with a "dedication" confirming that "the patrimony of Your Royal Highness toward my *Essays on Some Maladies of Angola* drove me again to ask Your Highness to protect these my writings. They are no less important than the former, which had the fortune to receive your approval."[39]

"The simplicity of principles is uniquely suitable to metaphysics and the abstract sciences"

In closing, we will highlight Azeredo's own final words.[40] The last years of his short life, which were spent as a physician at the Lisbon Royal Military Hospital in Xabregas (1801) and assigned as a physician to the Royal Chamber (1806), he dedicated to clinical work and writing.[41] He almost certainly worked from home, as was normal, and treated the "troops," and not for the first time.

His writing campaign resulted in two major unpublished titles, the aforementioned "Introduction to the Pathology of the Human Body" and "Collection of Clinical Observations," both of which contained dedications and signed prefaces. The former work is dated 1802, while the latter is undated but deals with actual cases that occurred in 1803.[42] In both we find Azeredo committed to a very particular legacy.

"Introduction to the Pathology of the Human Body" is an extended account of the successive impasses affecting systematic medical thought at the end of the eighteenth century. We now know how limited such perspectives were at the time. However, Azeredo's voice brings the contemporary testimony to life, providing a "clinical," almost surgical, view of the speculative standoff affecting all the "systematics" whom he listened to and studied, without closing the door to either science or philosophy. In the "Collection of Clinical Observations" he states, with redoubled conviction:

> The greatest advantage brought by the freedom of thought of our time is in the knowledge that the philosophical sciences should not be involved with the life sciences, and that it is only with a great deal of caution that the principles of mathematics, physics, chemistry, and of natural history should be applied to physiology and pathology. The laws of the animate body are very different from the laws of the inanimate body. While physicians explained themselves using the principles and rules of peripatetic, Cartesian, and mechanic philosophy, medicine was a slave to these sciences and the vital laws were unknown.

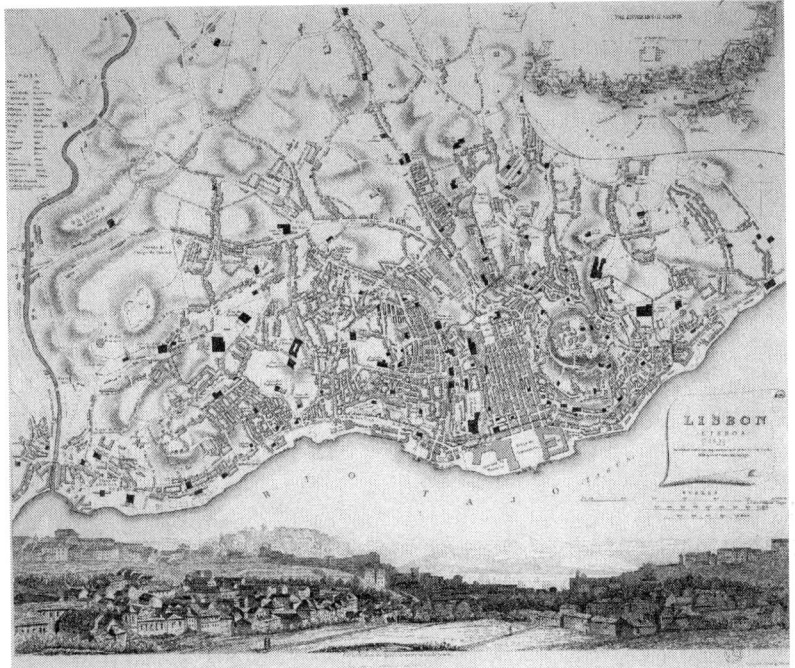

Lisbon, Portugal; overhead and horizon views, with the Bairro Alto neighborhood, where José Pinto de Azeredo lived out the final years of his life, visible. Engraving, J. Hershall, 1833. Published by Chapman & Hall, London, 1833.

Medicine is not a capricious science, and I run as far as possible from the hypotheses to contain medical philosophy within its true limits. I leave the physiologists to investigate whether galvanic fluid is, or is not, electric fluid; whether it is or is not nervous fluid; if it is or is not the cause of sensation and of movement. They may ask whether the active and sensitive atmosphere surrounding the nerves is, or is not, real, while I concern myself with the analysis of practical cases observed at the bedside of the ill. While they debate doctrines that are not yet well established, I study the man by studying within man himself.[43]

Because he was seriously ill, Azeredo did not follow the royal family to Brazil in 1807.[44] He was unable to fulfill his last wish: to return to the country in which he was born, to have some peace.

In 1805, at the age of forty-one, Azeredo made his brother his sole heir (perhaps in remembrance of the time when the two went to conquer Edinburgh together, and of the sibling who looked after him when he was still so young). On 15 April 1810 he died, with full sacrament, in the rua larga de São Roque, in Lisbon. Part of his legacy included his library, and some of the manuscripts inherited by his brother, destined, fortunately, to be held now in the Portuguese National Library.

PART TWO

Manuel Silvério Marques
(Centro de Filosofía da Universidade de Lisboa)

We believe Azeredo's life and work document and point to two key domains and historic principles: first, that a colonized "periphery" (in this case, Brazil) can achieve scientific and political ascendency over the colonial "center" (Portugal)—that necessity is the mother of invention, and distance dilutes sovereignty; and second, that the discontinuity thesis in the history (and philosophy) of the sciences appears to be corroborated by the growing dissociation of ideologies, doctrines, practices, technologies and/or (the then incipient and limited) medical utensils conditioning them—from precision scales to the microscope, the thermometer, right up to and including the scholarly journal—that occurred at the dawn of modern medicine. While we focus our attention in *Essays on Some Maladies of Angola*,[45] we refer to Azeredo's other works, along with earlier publications by others, as well as current research that touches on him. In Azeredo's time, the expanding Portuguese experience with diseases because of overseas exploration and colonization, as well as responses to the exigencies of war, advanced the means of promoting public health, and hygienism emerged. Azeredo's *Essays on Some Maladies of Angola* is a testament to this difficult—at times heroic—struggle for health in the tropics in the sociopolitical context of a Portuguese empire that was both weak (following the dismissal in 1777 of the "enlightened despot" the Marquês de Pombal) and ambivalent. This ambivalence was evident in the late baroque Basílica da Estrela (Queen Maria I's monumental response to Pombal's anticlericalism) and in the pseudo-romantic classicism of the Lisbon Opera, which stood in stark contrast to the liberalism manifested in the foundation, in 1779, of the Lisbon Academy of Sciences by the second Duke of Lafões — an academy that, by royal order, was permitted to publish without censorship.[46] In both Portugal and Brazil, opinion was divided between Anglophiles and Francophiles, between "conservatives" and those who embraced the foreign, and — to simplify — between progressives and reactionaries, "federalists" and "autonomists" (which were not entirely coincident parties and groupings). Angola at that time was a land where, in the words of a senior official, the ills of the "political and moral body" outweighed those of the physical body.[47] In effect, Luanda was a depository of slaves, ivory, wax, and seeds, and its largest market was Brazil. While the city had a more or less permanent population of approximately four thousand, annually there were around ten times as many slaves living and dying in transit. The time during which Martinho de Mello e Castro was minister for the overseas territories and of the navy was a period of opportunity and progress in natural and scientific philosophy. For example, for twenty years the Brazilian-born naturalist Joaquim José da Silva (who was, among other things, Angola's secretary-general from 1783 to 1808, and who was taught at the University of Coimbra by Domenico Vandelli) participated in and promoted important philosophical expeditions to the Angolan wilderness.[48]

A citizen of the Enlightenment, Azeredo was a polymath and, as far as we are aware, had mastered the laboratory skills of experimental chemistry. It is this fact, and the environment described above, that explain how the young physician was able to present the results of his important and well-received "Chemical Examination of the Atmosphere of Rio de Janeiro" (published in 1790) to the Literary Society of Rio de Janeiro in 1789.[49]

With the new *mathesis* (universal science), natural theology disappeared, natural philosophy changed radically, modern biology was born, and the number of theories and technologies multiplied in physics (e.g., electricity), chemistry (the discovery of oxygen), botany and pharmacology (opiates). Further, physiology (muscular and nervous irritability, motility, and sensitivity) developed, with the perfection of the thermometer, accurate scales, improved optics, and applied statistics. As Angola's physician general, Azeredo therefore lived through a period of rapid advances in the history of knowledge and the changes in its transmission, and of open conflict between the ideas of popular emancipation, a newly independent United States, the French Revolution, and European imperialism. His intellectual value was announced with his notable and pioneering 1790 analysis of Rio de Janeiro's atmosphere; it was also expressed in his *Magistral*—his inaugural address at the Luanda Royal Hospital on 11 September 1791.[50] It was then confirmed in the *Essays on Some Maladies of Angola* and in several unpublished works, including "Introduction to the Pathology of the Human Body"[51] and "Collection of Clinical Observations." We hope that the research currently being undertaken, especially in Brazil, will soon cast more light into the shadows and that the life and work of this Luso-Brazilian physician can be better known.

Who was José Pinto de Azeredo? How did he react to the events affecting him, from the 1789 Minas Gerais conspiracy (the so-called *Inconfidência*, an unsuccessful Brazilian independence movement) to the French Revolution? Did he, without fear or consequence, confront the great social transformations caused by nationalism in Europe and America? What religious faith did he embrace? What was his political ideology? Did he belong to any of the secret societies that proliferated within the more enlightened erudite circles? Within the positions that dominated in Portugal at that time, was he inclined to support the French party, the British party, or was he for neutrality?

He was a physician who followed closely the writings of Thomas Sydenham, Herman Boerhaave, Friedrich Hoffman, and William Cullen; who possessed the recently published *Dictionary of the Bunda Language* and the *Collection of Grammatica Observations on the Bunda Language* by Father Bernardo Maria de Cannecattim. Based on his last will and testament, wherein he nominated his brother as his sole heir, we know that at his death he had approximately 380 titles in his library.[52] The more theoretical texts suggest he was a devoted clinician—

one who was well educated and who kept abreast of scientific developments, a vigilant critic who took clear and vigorous positions: "I venture to say that more fevers are cured when they are completely ignored than are cured by bloodletting."[53] This reflective, objective, and prudential attitude is evident in the questions he asks, both of himself and of his readers, expressed with candor and frequency—that is, in the almost hyperbolic habit of questioning that is manifest in the *Essays* and, particularly, in his "Introduction to the Pathology of the Human Body." But is it legitimate to infer from the more practical narratives (such as the *Essays* and the clinical case reports) that he acted from conviction of the importance of the clinic, that he was moved not only by strict adherence to the Hippocratic lesson, but through his experience of the scientific limitations of empiricism? It is our conjecture that his praxis expressed, de jure, the renewed and "revolutionary" discourse of the "inner" or "visceral" man, endowed with an essential and clinically pregnant sensibility or *internal sense.*

We will seek to answer some of these questions and show that *Essays on Some Maladies of Angola* is a publication of great interest and value for medicine in Africa, and to prove that its author was a naturalist, a chemist, an anatomist who performed systematic autopsies, who had mastery of the microscope and, it could be said, was a forerunner of the scientific approach to the environment, health, and sickness, who was attentive toward people (and their language), to their sources of water, their air, and to their homes.[54]

He was parsimonious in his classification of infirmities and cautious in their treatment; he employed concepts that were then common, yet expressed great reserve for the dominant medical doctrines of the era: "This way of explaining nature's actions seems to me to be closest to the truth, and completely undermines the 'healing force of nature' [*medicatrix naturae*] that Cullen, without need, seeks to sustain."[55] He criticized Galenic medicine and promoted innovative ideas, from fibrillation theory to the beginnings of the notion of reflex (Thomas Willis), of irritability and of *incitability*.[56] He was an opponent of medical simplification and speculation, especially that of John Brown.[57] He often mentions the cellular, weblike substance (*tela celulosa*),[58] and the tissues and cells found here and there; yet he read Bichat, and did not suspect, as the majority of his contemporaries did, the meaning and explanatory potential of cellular theory. His medicine was yet that of miasmas, before the discovery and demonstration of microorganisms, of their existence or of the fermentation and pathology resulting from them.[59]

As pertinent as it may be, we will not discuss the role of the military and civilian medical institutions, the welfare institutions in continental Portugal and the overseas territories — bodies, moreover, that held informal classes in medicine throughout the empire. Nor will we examine the historiography of tropical medicine and health in the army, or in the navy. Some themes and selected controversies in the historiography of modern medicine faced by Azeredo will be mentioned schematically at the end, where we see that he was an adversary of the nosography of fevers that was prevalent at the time.

The Theory and Practice of "Tropical Medicine"

Essays is a very personal and mature reflection on the treatment of tropical fevers in comparison to European maladies. Perhaps Azeredo's most decisive choice was the abandonment of the idea of plethora and of evacuation (including bloodletting), and his notion that the "fevers of Angola are of the same nature as those . . . observed in other countries situated in the Torrid Zone. . . . The paroxysms, the crises, the progress and the symptoms are all the same, and for this the methods of curing them I am about to describe must be the same as those applied to fevers in other climates."[60]

In the tropics, according to Manuel Fernandes Nabuco, Francisco Mello Franco, and the young José Pinto de Azeredo, a good semiology is very important: pulse, respiration, face, signs of suppuration or putrefaction, hydration and the texture of the tongue — in that order; the internal organs, particularly the liver, also must be evaluated.[61] In the *Essays*, Azeredo specifically highlighted some universal therapeutic principles, the raison d'être of which were only centuries later determined: the rejection of bloodletting and of poly-pharmacotherapy; the frequent ingestion of liquids (saline solutions); light meals; the control of hypothermia, of dryness, of pains, and digestive disorders. His view on drugs was not so original: he was an advocate of the early and sparing prescription of active drugs—quinine, nux vomica, white arsenic, and coconut bark for intermittent fevers,[62] and tartar emetic, opium, and quinine for remittent fevers—all the time attentive to the purity and activity of the Galenic preparations, to the organism's reaction and the verification of results (outcomes). Consequently, Azeredo used available pharmaceuticals, measuring their effect by the symptomatic response to high doses of quinine, opium, arsenic, antimony, and other active substances.[63]

In his book *A History of Medicine in Portugal*, Maximiano Lemos quite rightly called attention to the significant number of Luso-Brazilians who studied medicine in Europe, at Coimbra, Paris, Edinburgh, Montpellier, etc., during the eighteenth and nineteenth centuries.[64] It is worthwhile to quickly analyze a sample. He highlights the fact that, like Francisco Mello Franco and others, José Pinto de Azeredo discussed the value of the neo-methodist doctrine that was both popular and dominant during the time of Brown; however, while Azeredo rejected it on principle, adopting stimulation therapy (based on quinine) for fevers, Mello Franco, following Cullen, opted for anti-phlogistics.[65] This is explained comparatively in the table below.[66]

Unlike Cullen or Azeredo, the Brunonians prescribed general measures, such as sthenics or tonics for fever.[67] However, this was based on a "physiology" that was too simplistic and frequently wrong.[68] Additionally, Azeredo certainly denounced the concept of phlogistic diathesis,[69] which had obvious consequences for the treatment of febrile symptoms and was seriously concerned with measuring temperatures with a new tool that was then entering into the nurse's routine: the mercury thermometer.[70]

Some Controversial Topics:

A) Fever

Fever is plural and heterogeneous: complaint, epiphenomenon, reaction, symptom, syndrome, and illness. The chapter on the nosography of fevers is, for Azeredo, a theme of little clinical importance: unlike Cullen and the majority of his colleagues, he was not interested in the "botanic," Linnaean, or any other classification of fevers:

Medical doctrine and practice of
several Brazilian contemporaries of J. P. Azeredo

	Scot.*	Irritab.**	Therapy of fevers	Blood-letting	Scientific profile
J. M. Chaves	No	Yes, anti-solidism	Anti-phlogistic & anti-gastric & stimulant	Yes	Good studies on agues and quinine use; orthodox view on fevers
F. M. Franco	No	Yes, qualified	Anti-phlogistic & anti-gastric; stimulant?	Yes	"Scientific tropical" medicine; hygienist; against Brunism
J. P. Azeredo	Yes	Yes	Stimulant +/- quinine	No	Chemical experiments; criticism of phlogistic diathesis & of medical systems
B. A. Gomes	Yes	Yes	Anti-phlogistic & stimulant	No?	Scientific medicine; research of Brazilian flora
H. X. Baeta	Yes	Yes	Anti-phlogistic & anti-gastric; stimulant	Yes	Translated Erasmus, Darwin works; orthodox view on fevers

*Scottish studies
**Irritability doctrine; bloodletting prescription

The old physicians, and even some modern ones, have introduced so many different kinds of continuous fevers that the study of them is tiresome and almost incomprehensible. There just needs to be one more symptom, or the fever just needs be more serious, for them to create a new type of fever, even when both its cause and its treatment are the same. . . . Laborious and confident observation is the only way to learn how to seek the methods most suitable for the treatment of the illness, and from those particular facts we will, like Bacon, assess the general effects of the proximate cause and decide on the treatment to be administered in order to obtain a cure.[71]

Nevertheless, Azeredo distinguished the pyrexias, the "real" or primary fevers, from the inflammations, phlegmasia, or symptomatic fevers that "have periods of when their severity abates, even if only brief or unobserved. Thus we can say that, with the exception of symptomatic pyrexias, there are no fevers that can truly be called continuous. Therefore all fevers are either intermittent or remittent."[72]

> The *pyrexia* resulting from topical affections is not a primary complaint, but rather is a symptom of the affection, and is therefore not a fever. There are no inflammatory fevers, because all inflammation causes local affection, of which the pyrexia is a symptom. If there is no topical blemish in the pyrexia, even though the pulse is strong and regular, the face flushed and red and without inflammation, this is because these symptoms do not always indicate it, nor are they enough to decide on the nature of the *phlogistic diathesis.*[73]

These were his preliminary considerations and definitions. Here we will not develop Michel Foucault's provocative insight of an absence, of something "unspoken" in relation to fevers that is associated, correctly we believe, to the struggle of the local versus the global, of the illness of the organ versus a general or (multi-) systemic illness; in other words, the clinical conflict: topical pyrexia or phlegmasia versus fever. This "polarization" is further complicated with the description and knowledge (of "slow" and chronic evolution) of the febrile illnesses of the tropics.

B) About dysentery and "tetanus"

In addition to the fevers (infectious) that, as we know today, accompany gastroenteritis, colitis, or diarrhea, Azeredo describes other processes associated with intestinal parasites; that is, the dysenteries that are very common in the tropics, and which nowadays are recognized as ameobic. His statements are blunt:

> There is nothing that can cast a clearer light and provide a more perfect idea of the proximate cause of dysentery than the dissection of corpses. . . . On dissecting a section of the colon and performing a detailed examination of its tunics [membranes], the nature of the complaint becomes clear. In it we find tubercles [lesions] in the form of pustules that appear in varying amounts and in different states. . . . In the muscular tunic I noted some small ulcers between the tubercles,

which were only discovered after taking care to clean out the mucus and bile, of which there is a great deal.[74]

As one contemporary physician and authority on medical history, Dr. João David de Morais, has noted, this passage signaled the end of empiricism and the beginning of scientific medicine in Portugal and Brazil.[75]

As for the convulsive conditions and the "tetanus," the situation is so much more complex and controversial. Azeredo displays a surprising and, in our view, incredible optimism, at least if we are to take what he wrote literally: "Now I can boast that I have found an excellent method of treating tetanus, one that has always produced good results."[76] There are no statements from independent observers; on the other hand, the data are so detailed and "frightening" that we can reject the idea that they were the result of self-delusion of the author, who, moreover, is not suspected of falsifying the evidence (if scholars once doubted that Azeredo knew and followed Brown's method, as we suspect, or that he had "copied" the recipe for large doses of opium "discovered" by Nabuco, these doubts have abated).[77] However, as David de Morais also notes, many of these cases were the convulsions of remittent (or intermittent) fevers that were cured with the administration of quinine, and not with mercury or opium; in other words, they were examples of cerebral malaria (and we must not exclude other common causes in that context, such as metabolic and ionic disorders).[78] Nevertheless, we must qualify this: surgical cleanliness and mercurial rubs may be effective during the *local* phase of infection by *Chlostridium tetani* and others (that is to say, during the toxin's preinvasive phase); opium is useful as a sedative. We know that thorough debridement and cleansing, including of the section of the nerve fibers of all patients suspected of having tetanus, and the generous application of the best chemical antiseptic of the day—mercury—could prevent or slow the progression of some types of tetanus before the spread of toxins throughout the nervous system. And as Morais notes, in those days the classic and optimal treatment for spasms and convulsion was the administration of (almost) unlimited doses of opium.[79]

Spasm of an *Imperium*

Despite the "gigantism" and the difficulties, which were considerable, in the period that included the reign of Queen Maria I, Portugal made great efforts to develop in the arts and industries, to establish frontiers and exploit the riches of its overseas territories: philosophical voyages and military expeditions were planned and executed with greater or lesser degrees of success. At that time Angola was under the hegemonic domination of Brazil, and the African population was hideously exploited by the Europeans and others.

Who in Angola were the patients of José Pinto de Azeredo and his colleagues and students? We must assume that they were predominantly free Luandans (the majority), some poor whites who were often *degredados* (Portuguese convicts forced to emigrate to the colonies—this group formed a significant proportion of the European elite in Africa, both then and later); free and enslaved mixed-race peoples; freed and enslaved blacks from Luanda; and, while in transit, servants of the Crown, members of expeditionary forces, sailors, and people from the Angolan interior. They were people of many different social statuses, cultures, and ethnicities, as was the case on the other side of the Atlantic traffic. Apparently Azeredo did not exclude anyone, and explicitly mentions the "black people" and the "many white children of the country," the Europeans, the Brazilians, and perhaps also the many slaves.[80] Did he not rather pointedly note elsewhere that "human nature was and always will be the same for all time and in every nation"?[81]

Our tropical physician left a very clear and pragmatic message: fever in the tropics is such an emergency that the traditional wait for the crisis would risk the loss of the opportunity for a cure. All the symptoms are important because they soon "grow to become mortal," which is something everyone should fear.[82]

Our limited goal was to present the main contours of our knowledge of the man, of his personal and professional biography, and of his encounter with the emerging sciences and contemporary medical systems on three Atlantic continents. José Pinto de Azeredo frequented the great classics of science and philosophy, from Hippocrates to Newton, from Cicero to Rousseau. He subscribed to *Philosophical Transactions*, was familiar with the microscopic observations of Leeuwenhoek, of Hooke, of Swammerdam, and of Gleichen-Russworm. He knew of the pathographies of Malpighi and Morgan (particularly the *Dissertationes medicas* and *De sedis morboram*), of Buffon's natural history and Wolff and Spallanzani's studies on reproduction. He mastered the experiments of Priestley and Black on air, and those of Scheele and Lavoisier on *caloric* (that is, heat, understood as a chemical element) and the chemistry of oxygen. He was aware of Galvani's electrical fluids and understood the theory of atoms and the use of the thermometer better than many of his colleagues who had the privilege to see his work published during their lifetimes. This is a sketch of the story of a physician of whom we know very little, but who, through his texts, and repelled by the rigidity of medical systems, demonstrated innovative methodologies, searched for the contradictory, adopted the practices of rigorously citing sources and clearly explaining his doubts, his ignorance, and his uncertainties, but who did not fail to describe his experience and the rationale governing his medical and philosophical decisions.

Notes

We would like to acknowledge the important contributions made by Teresa Saraiva and Isabel Abecasis of the Torre do Tombo national archive, Dr. Júlio Rodrigues da Costa of the Oporto Municipal Public Library, and the physicians João David de Morais and Joaquim Barradas to the composition of this short professional and intellectual biography of José Pinto de Azeredo.

1. Emílio Joaquim da Silva Maia, "Elogio histórico do Dr. José Pinto de Azeredo," *Revista Trimestral de História e Geografia ou Jornal do Instituto Histórico e Geográfico Brasileiro*, tomo 2, supplement to no. 8 (1840), pp. 59–66.

2. We believe this refers to José de Rezende Costa, son of captain José de Rezende Costa, who was born at the Arraial da Laje, Vila de São José do Rio das Mortes, Minas Gerais, in 1765, and who died on 17 June 1841.

3. Maia, 59–66. The chronological references in this text are almost entirely in error. Azeredo was not born in 1763; he did not graduate in 1787; he did not return to Lisbon in 1792; and he did not die in 1807.

4. Azeredo's baptism certificate, Arquivo Nacional da Torre do Tombo (ANTT), *Feitos Findos, Inventário de Bens, letra* I, J, *maço* 194, nr. 7 (folios not numbered).

5. Ibid.

6. Manuel Serrano Pinto, Marco Antonio G. Cecchini, Isabel Maria Malaquias, Lycia Maria Moreira-Nordemann, and João Rui Pita, "O médico brasileiro José Pinto de Azeredo (1766?–1810) e o exame químico da atmosfera do Rio de Janeiro," in *Manguinhos—História, Ciências, Saúde* (Rio de Janeiro: FIOCRUZ, 2005) 12:3, pp. 617–73.

7. ANTT, *Feitos Findos, Inventário de Bens, letra* I, J, *maço* 194, nr. 7 (folios not numbered).

8. Ibid.

9. Maia, p. 61.

10. Pinto et al. (2005), p. 620.

11. For more on the beginnings of Silva Alvarenga's school in Rio in 1782 (probably in August) see Gustavo Henrique Tuna, *Silva alvarenga representante das Luzes na América portuguesa* (doctoral thesis, department of history, Universidade de São Paulo, 2009), pp. 76, 164.

12. Áurea Adão, *Estado absoluto e ensino das primeiras letras: As escolas régias (1772–1794)* (Lisbon: Fundação Calouste Gulbenkian, 1997), pp. 221–22, 325.

13. Maia, p. 61.

14. This is how they appear in the register of the University of Edinburgh. See Pinto et al. (2005), p. 621. For more on how easily people changed their names during the early modern period see Martha Daisson Hameister, "Uma contribuição ao estudo da onomástica no período colonial: Os nomes e o povoamento do extremo Sul da Colônia (Continente do Rio Grande de São Pedro, c. 1735–c. 1777)," in *Temas setecentistas: Governos e populações no império português*, ed. Antonio César de Almeida Santos and Andréa Doré (Curitiba: UFPR-SCHLA / Fundação Araucária, 2008), pp. 459–78.

15. See Pinto et al. (2005), p. 621.

16. Alexander Bower, *The History of the University of Edinburgh: Chiefly Compiled from Original Papers and Records, Never Before Published*, vol. 3 (Edinburgh: Oliphant, Waugh and Innes, 1830), 103–10; Alexander Grant, *The Story of the University of Edinburgh during the First Three Hundred Years*, vol. 1 (London: Longmans, Green and Co., 1884), pp. 320, 330–31; John Dixon Comrie, *History of Scottish Medicine to 1860* (London: Ballière, Tindall and Cox, 1927), pp. 199, 202–16.

17. Bower, ibid.; Grant, ibid.; Comrie, ibid.

18. This appears in José Pinto de Azeredo, "Isagòge pathologica do corpo humano dedicada a Sua Alteza Real o Principe Regente Nosso Senhor" (manuscript, dated 1802), BNP, *códice* 8482, f. 355. An annotated edition of this manuscript has been published as José Pinto de Azeredo, *Isagòge pathologica do corpo humano*, ed. António Braz de Oliveira and Manuel Silvério Marques (Lisbon: Colibri, 2014).

19. Andrew Duncan, *Medical Commentaries . . . Exhibiting a Concise View of the Latest and Most Important Discoveries in Medicine and Medical Philosophy*, vol. 3 (Edinburgh: C. Elliot and T. Kay, 1789), p. 396.

20. Joseph Black, *Essays and Observations, Physical and Literary, Read before a Society in Edinburgh and Published by Them*, vol. 2 (Edinburgh: G. Hamilton and J. Balfour, 1756), pp. 157–225.

21. José Pinto de Azeredo, "Exame quimico da atmosphera do Rio de Janeiro," in *Jornal Encyclopédico* (Lisbon: Antonio Rodrigues Galhardo, Março 1790), 281. See also Pinto et al. (2005), pp. 622, 658.

22. Gulielmus Cullen, *Synopsis nosologiae methodicae exhibens* (Edinburgh: Prostant venales apud Gulielmum Creech, 1780).

23. That is, the Roman Methodist (or Methodic) school of physicians, active during the first century BCE, who formulated some of the most influential doctrines of medicine within the Roman Empire.

24. Azeredo, "Isagòge" (1802), manuscript p. 47. Letter (b) indicates a footnote that says "Vej. Jone's inquir."—that is, see Robert Jones, *An Inquiry into the State of Medicine on the Principles of Inductive Philosophy* (Edinburgh: T. Longman and T. Cadell, 1781).

25. In the brothers' individual records at the University of Edinburgh the only mention is RMS-1786 (Royal Medical Society, 1786).

26. Note that Leiden's regulations allowed for the conclusion of medical courses in only two years. See Bower, 217, in which he cites Charles Goodale; also Grant; Comrie; and Gerrit Arie Lindeboom, "Medical Education in the Netherlands, 1575–1750," in *History of Medical Education*, ed. Charles Donald O'Malley (Berkeley: University of California Press, 1968), pp. 203, 213–14.

27. *Dissertatio medica inauguralis de Podagra. Quam annuente summo numime. . . . Eruditorum examini submittit Josephus Pinto ab Azeredo, Brasiliensis, Soc. Reg. Med. Edin. Soc. Phys. Amer. Edin, Soc. & Praeses Annuus. Ad Diem XI. Junii MDC-CLXXXVIII. . . .* Only a detailed examination of the thesis will show if Azeredo mentions the controversy surrounding the treatment of gout in the wake of the Brunist principles and therapeutic methods. See Günter B. Risse and Ramunas Kondratas, "Brunonianism in Britain and Europe," *Medical History* 8 (1988): pp. 46–62, 78–88.

28. In Latin, *definition, historia, causae remotae, causa proxima,* and *ratio medendi.* The mention on the graduation register is from Philip Christiaan Molhuysen, *Bronnen tot de Geschiedenis der Leidsche Universiteit* (The Hague: Martinus Nijhoff, 1913–24), vol. 6, pp. 123–24.

29. "Patente de Sua Majestade em que faz mercê ao Doutor José Pinto de Azeredo de físico mor deste Reino de Angola," *Arquivos de Angola* [Iª série], vol. 4, nr. 41–48, pp. 149–50, Luanda, May–December 1938; Pinto et al. (2005), p. 628. It is not clear that Azeredo had received a grant or benefited from royal patronage in order to study in a foreign country.

30. See Pinto et al. (2005), p. 621.

31. ANTT, Chancelarias Régias, D. Maria I, *livro* 32, p. 323, cited in Pinto et al. (2005), p. 624, and p. 653, n. 6.

32. *Jornal enciclopédico dedicado á Rainha N. Senhora, e destinado para instrução geral com a notícia dos novos descobrimentos em todas as ciências, e artes* (Lisbon: Oficina de António Rodrigues Galhardo, July 1779–May 1793). The "Chemical Examination" was discussed in detail in Pinto et al. (2005), which includes a facsimile of this publication.

33. José Pinto de Azeredo, *Ensaios sobre algumas enfermidades de Angola* (Lisbon:

Regia Officina Typografica, 1799), p. vii. A new annotated edition of this book has just come out in Portugal: José Pinto de Azeredo, *Ensaios sobre algumas enfermidades de Angola*, ed. António Braz de Oliveira and Manuel Silvério Marques (Lisbon: Colibri, 2013).

34. Manuel Ruela Pombo, "Bando sobre a abertura da aula, de medicina e anatomia," *Diogo Cão* 1, 5 (1932): 169–70, and republished in *Arquivos de Angola* 4, nos. 41–48 (May–December 1938), pp. 165–66; *Arquivos de Angola* 9, nos. 35–36 (2nd series, January–June 1952), pp. 23–24. The term *bando* (in English, "band") was used to describe any public notice or proclamation that was to be made by a town crier.

35. José Pinto de Azeredo, "Oração de Sapiência feita e recitada no dia 11 de Setembro de 1791" (manuscript, 1791), BNP, *códice* 8486//1, f. 3r.

36. See Azeredo's petition dated 1805 in the Arquivo Histórico Ultramarino, Portugal Collection, Rio de Janeiro, box 223, document 71.

37. From the time of Azeredo's stay in Angola (1791–97), we have the manuscripts of "Anatomia dos ossos, e vasos lymphaticos do corpo. . . ." (manuscript, Lisbon, 1791), BNP, *códice* 8485//2, ff. 77–87; "Apontamentos de matéria e química médicas" (manuscript, 1791–97), BNP, *códice* 8484, f. 107; "Apontamentos de medicina" (manuscript, no date), BNP, *códex* 8485//1, ff. 1–76v.; "Estudos anatómicos" (manuscript, no date), BNP, *códice* 8486//2, ff. 8–20v.; "Observação geral sobre as laxaçoens" (manuscript, no date), BNP, *códice* 8486//4, ff. 90–98v.; "Prolegomenos da myologia" (manuscript, no date), BNP *códice* 8486//3, ff. 21–89v.; "Prolegomenos sobre as glândulas" (manuscript, no date), BNP, *códice* 8485//3, ff. 88–92v.; and "Tratado anatómico dos ossos, vasos linfáticos, e glândulas" (manuscript, no date), BPMP, *códice* 1126.

38. See José Pinto de Azeredo, "Ensaios sobre algumas enfermidades d'Angola. Dedicados ao sereníssimo D. João Príncipe do Brasil por José Pinto de Azeredo" (manuscript, 1799), 4 f., 112 p. ANTT, PT/TT/RMC/B-E/001/1858.

39. The dedication is contained, word for word, in the dedications of "Isagòge pathologica do corpo humano" and in the "Collecção de observaçoens clinicas" (manuscript, post-1803), BNP, *códice* 8483, f. 1r.

40. Azeredo, "Prefação," *in* "Collecção" (post-1803), f. 3v.

41. Pinto et al. (2005), pp. 633–35.

42. BNP, *códice* 8482 and 8483, respectively. In the "Isagòge" manuscript there is a title page dated 1802. The "Collecção de observaçoens clinicas" has no title page; the date is therefore attributed.

43. Azeredo, "Collecção," f. 5v.–6r.

44. Pinto et al. (2005), p. 636.

45. Azeredo, *Ensaios* (1799).

46. See BNP Special Collections, *códice* 3370, a volume of diverse administrative papers of the Academia Real das Ciências de Lisboa, including *Breves Instrucções aos correspondentes . . . sobre história, da natureza* (dated 1781) (Lisbon: Regia Officina Typografia, 1812), pp. 66–68; and José Alberto Teixeira Rebelo da Silva, "A Academia Real das Ciências de Lisboa (1779–1834): Ciências e hibridismo numa periferia europeia" (doctoral thesis: Universidade de Lisboa, Faculdade de Ciências [Secção Autónoma de História e Filosofia das Ciências], 2015), p. 31.

47. For the statistics see Ilídio Amaral, *Luanda: Estudo de geografia urbana* (Lis-

bon: Tipografia Atlântida Editora, 1968), pp. 49–51. In 1791 the governor of Angola, Dom Manuel de Almeida e Vasconcellos, communicated the following to the Overseas Council: "Experience has always done justice to the bad reputation of this climate; moreover its diseases, morals and politics do, in my opinion, exceed all those that influence the physical body." Cited in Amaral, p. 48.

48. William J. Simon, *Scientific Expeditions in the Portuguese Overseas Territories (1783–1808)* (Lisbon: Instituto de Investigação Científica Tropical, 1983), pp. 79–104, 155–67.

49. Pinto et al. (2005), pp. 650, 653; Azeredo, "Exame químico" (1790), pp. 259–88.

50. José Pinto de Azeredo, "Oração de Sapiência feita e recitada no dia 11 de Setembro de 1791" (manuscript, 1791), BNP, *códice* 8486, f. 3r.

51. The Portuguese title is "Isagòge patológica do corpo humano dedicada a Sua Alteza Real o Principe Regente Nosso Senhor," a manuscript Azeredo composed in 1802.

52. Marques and Oliveira (2011), pp. 139, 148.

53. Azeredo, *Ensaios* (1799), p. 79.

54. Ibid., p. 36.

55. Ibid., pp. 35–36.

56. Ibid., pp. 30–31: "It was enough for Baglivi to prove the action of moving fibers as the engines of the animated body, for physicians to return their attention to the movement of solids and to stop believing in the existence of a viscous fluid, or *lentor*, within the extremities of the small vessels in which the fever originates."

57. Günter B. Risse, "Brunonian Therapeutics: New Wine on Old Bottles," *Medical History*, Supplement 8 (1988): pp. 46–62; and Ramunas Kondratas, "The Brunonian Influence on the Medical Thought and Practice of Joseph Frank," *Medical History*, Supplement 8 (1988): pp. 75–88.

58. Albrecht von Haller, *Physiology: Being a Course of Lectures upon the Visceral Anatomy and Vital Oeconomy of Human Bodies. . . .* 2 vols. (London: printed for W. Innys and J. Richardson, 1754), vol. 1, p. 16; and Haller, *Élémens de physiologie. . . .* (French translation from Latin by M. Toussaint Bordenave) (Paris: Chez Guillyn, 1769), pp. 3, 5, 7; 140–44; and Haller, *Prima linea physiologiae in usum praelectionum academicarum* (Göttingen: Apud A. Vandennoeck, 1751), p. 13.

59. Bruno Latour, *Guerre et paix des microbes* (Paris: La Découverte, 2001), pp. 59, 132.

60. Azeredo, *Ensaios* (1799), p. vii.

61. Manuel Fernandes Nabuco, "Observaçoens medico-chi[r]urgicas, anatomicas: Unicas até os nossos tempos, nas quaes se demonstra até onde tenho chegado com adossis [*sic*] do opio tebaico, em substancia; e laudano liquido, para serem assistidas as contracçoens convulsivas rezultadas das feridas, e chagas mais acontecimentos ofensivos e poderem de hoje em diante servir de guia no exercicio curatorio aos professores da Medicina Cirurgical. . . ." (manuscript, Bahia, Brazil, dated 15 November 1785), BNP, *códice* 11241, f. 189.

62. Azeredo claimed a pioneering role for the use of coconut bark, which seems to be confirmed in Joseph-François-Xavier Sigaud, *Du climat et des maladies du Brésil* (Paris: Chez Fortin, Masson et Compagnie Libraires, 1844), pp. 130, 247. The

properties of coconut (not specifically its bark) were described by Garcia de Orta in *Dialogue* 16 of *Coloquio dos simples e drogas he cousas medicinais da Índia.* . . . (Goa: Ioannes de Endem, 1563), which was then adapted by Cristovão da Costa in chapter 14 of *Tractado de las drogas y medicinas de las Indias orientales* (Burgos, Spain: Martin de Victoria, 1578). It is interesting to note that, according to Eric Brossard, coconut continues to be used in Angolan Umbundo medicine today; see Eric Brossard, *La médecine traditionnel au centre et à l'ouest de l'Angola* (Lisbon: Instituto de Investigações Científica Tropical, 1996), pp. 55, 239, and 320.

63. J. J. R. Fraústo da Silva and R. J. P. Williams, *The Biological Chemistry of the Elements: The Inorganic Chemistry of Life* (Oxford: Oxford University Press, 1993), pp. 531–52. It is known that antimony is both a febrifuge and an antiparasitic that is particularly effective against schistosomiasis. Azeredo, *Ensaios* (1799), pp. 61, 70, and 77. To contrast this with the traditional antiphlogistic method of aggressive bloodletting practiced by Benjamin Rush, for example, in yellow fever, see Kenneth R. Foster, Mary F. Jenkins, and Anna Coxe Toogood, "The Philadelphia Yellow Fever," in *Scientific American*, 279:2 (August 1998), pp. 68–73.

64. Maximiano de Lemos, *História de medicina em Portugal: Doutrinas e instituições*, 2 vols. (Lisbon: Editora Dom Quixote and Ordem dos Médicos, 1991), vol. 2, pp. 232, 249, 251. Lemos insists that the most popular "systems" in Portugal and Brazil were those of the Scottish physician William Buchan (1729–1805) and of Brown, followed by that of Cullen.

65. Bruno Barreiros, "O discurso higienista no Portugal do século XVIII: Tradição e modernidade," in *Arte Médica e Imagem do Corpo* (Lisbon: Biblioteca Nacional de Portugal, 2010), pp. 123–36.

66. José Manuel Chaves (1746–1821), *Febriologia accomodada também para as pessoas curiosas conforme a observação na praxe de 20 anos tem feito José Manuel Chaves, médico do partido de* Condeixa (Coimbra: Real Oficina da Universidade, 1790); José Manuel Chaves, *Elementos de medicina practica* (Lisbon: Regia Typographia Silviana, 1792), a Portuguese translation of the fourth and final English-language edition of William Cullen's *Practice of Medicine* by Dr. Édouard-François-Marie Bosquillon (2 vols.) (Paris: 1785–87), using a French-language version translated by José Manuel Chaves; Francisco Mello Franco (1757–1823), *Ensaio sobre as febres com observação analytica à sua topographia, clima e demais particularidades que influi no caracter das febres do Rio de Janeiro* (Lisbon: Typographia da Real Academia das Ciências, 1829); Francisco Mello Franco, *Elementos de hygiene, ou dictames theoreticos, e practicos para conservar a saude, e prolongar a vida*, 2nd ed, (Lisbon: Academia Real das Ciências, 1819); Bernardino António Gomes (1768–1823), *Memória sobre a* Ipecacuanha fusca *do Brasil ou cipó das nossas boticas* (Lisbon: Typographia Calcographica do Arco do Cego, 1801); Bernardino António Gomes, *Método de curar a febre tifóide ou as febres malignas contagiosas pela ablução de água fria.* . . . (Lisbon: Typopgraphia da Real Academia das Sciencias, 1812); Henrique Xavier Baeta (1776–1854), *Dissertatio medica inaugurale de thypho* (Edinburgh: G. Stewart and Society, Academic Typographer, 1800); Henrique Xavier Baeta, *Dissertatio de febris intermittentibus princ. Medendis* (Edinburgh: J. Pillans and Son, 1800); Henrique Xavier Baeta, *Comparative View of the Theories and Practice of Drs. Cullen, Brown, and Darwin, in the Treatment of Fever, and Acute*

Rheumatism (London: Luke Hansard, for J. Johnson, 1800); Henrique Xavier Baeta, *Memória sobre a febre contagiosa que grassou em Lisboa desde outubro de 1810 até agosto de 1811* (Lisbon: Impressão Régia, 1812). Note: a recent investigation of matriculation records at Edinburgh University has not been able to confirm that Bernardino A. Gomes pursued medical studies there (an assertion based on references made in Gomes's own publications); but such records are incomplete.

67. Sigaud did not share this interpretation.

68. Azeredo, *Ensaios* (1799), pp. 33–34. What Brown called "asthenia," Cullen called "debility" and "atonia." See W. F. Bynum and Vivian Nutton, eds., *Theories of Fever from Antiquity to the Enlightenment* (London: Wellcome Institute for the History of Medicine, 1981; *Medical History* Supplement no. 1), p. 143.

69. For Cullen's theories on phlogistic diathesis see William Cullen, *First Lines of the Practice of Physics* (Edinburgh: Printed for C. Elliott and T. Cadell, 1784), section 247, p. 225; and Cullen, *Works, Containing His Physiology, Nosology, and the First Lines of the Practice of Physic; With Numerous Extracts from His Manuscript Papers, and from His Treatise of the Materia Medica*, 2 vols. (Edinburgh: W. Blackwood, 1827), vol. 2, p. 7. However, in his "Isagòge," Azeredo makes use of such concepts as asthenic, inflammatory, and phlogistic diathesis; see Azeredo, "Isagòge" (1802), pp. 32, 54, 80, 207.

70. Quoting Gomes Pereira and Francis Bacon (who showed that temperature is distinguished only by intensity) and Swedish apothecary Carl Wilhelm Scheele, who showed experimentally the importance of oxygen in the air for combustion, and using Santorio's thermometer, "which demonstrated that heat in any form has the effect of dilating the body," Azeredo once again showed himself to be methodologically current and rigorous, by insisting on the research of the Scottish physician Georges Martine (1702–41) in relation to thermometers, and was careful in his choice of medical instruments. See Azeredo, "Isagòge" (1802), p. 198.

71. Azeredo, *Ensaios* (1799), p. 4. In his *First Lines of the Pratica of Physic*, William Cullen classifies pyrexias into five groups: fevers, inflammations, eruptions, hemorrhage, and flows; Cullen (1784 [1827]), section 7, p. 8.

72. Azeredo, *Ensaios* (1799), p. 3.

73. Ibid., p. 2.

74. Ibid., p. 107.

75. João David de Morais, personal correspondence with Manuel Marques, during 2013–14.

76. Azeredo, *Ensaios* (1799), p. 143. It is worth noting that the extreme effectiveness of mercury as a local antiseptic meant that it was commonly used at home and in hospitals until quite recently (although like arsenic it is highly toxic, it is less easily absorbed through the skin); see Guido Majno, *The Healing Hand: Man and Wound in the Ancient World* (Cambridge, MA: Harvard University Press, 1975), pp. 153, 256; and Silva and Williams (1993), pp. 537–39.

77. Kondratas, "Brunonian Influence" (1988), pp. 75–88.

78. Compare with Azeredo, "Isagòge" (1802), pp. 102–10, 225. See also João David de Morais et al., "Subsídios para o conhecimento médico e antropológico do povo

Undulo; I: Estudos clínico-nutricional, parasitológico e sócio-epidemiológico de um grupo de crianças," *Anais do Instituto de Higiene e Medicina Tropical* 2:1–4 (1975), pp. 143–256.

79. Azeredo, *Ensaios* (1799), pp. 142–49. This therapeutic system is also used by Nabuco, as we have noted; see Nabuco (1785), f. 189; and Majno, pp. 198, 370, 414.

80. Azeredo, *Ensaios* (1799), pp. 52–53, 59. This hypothesis requires verification; but the truth is, it conforms to Azeredo's rationalist and pre-positivist ethos that devalued, on principle, the popular and traditional medicine that, at least in the case of uses for coconut, he had studied.

81. The quotation is from Azeredo's manuscript text "Oração de sapiência" that records a presentation given in Luanda, Angola, on 11 September 1791, cited in Azeredo, *Ensaios sobre algumas enfermidades d'Angola*, ed. Mário Milheiros (Luanda: Instituto de Investigação Científica de Angola, 1967), p. 14. The entire text of "Oração de sapiência" appears in José Pinto de Azeredo, *Tratado anatómico dos ossos, vasos lymphaticos e glândulas*, ed. Júlio Rodrigues da Costa (Lisbon: Colibri, 2014), pp. 13–24.

82. Azeredo, *Ensaios* (1799), p. 61.

ESSAYS ON

SOME MALADIES
OF ANGOLA

Dedicated to his Most Serene Majesty
Dom João, Prince of Brazil

BY

José Pinto de Azeredo,

Knight of the Order of Christ
Doctor of Medicine and Member
of Various Academies of Europe

LISBON

The Royal Typography Office

MDCCXCIX [1799]

Licensed under the authority of the Tribunal of the Royal Court

To his Most Serene Majesty Dom João, Prince of Brazil,

My Lord,

If I do not fear exposing myself to the censorship of critics with this small work that I now present to the public, it is because I hope it will be protected by the name of Your Highness. Only a patron as great as a prince whose breast heaves with love and the desire for his people's happiness can encourage me, sir, to debut as an Author and subject myself to vitriol. This compendium contains no more than the result of my experiences in discovering the swiftest means of attacking the diseases of a country as ailing as Angola, where I served as the Physician General.[1] I hope Your Highness will safeguard my vigilant observations and receive my offer as the highest token of my gratitude. While I may not deserve to be called a knowledgeable writer, I have always been a dutiful physician who wished to be useful to my fellow countrymen. While I am not able to heighten Your Highness's glory, my wish is that this work will at least serve to demonstrate to the world the love the Portuguese have for their Prince. May Lusitania count your triumphs through a long series of many days to come! May all the sovereigns in the universe, in all humanity, imitate in tranquil peace Your Highness's happy government! And may the sciences that Your Highness has raised anew celebrate your Highness's virtues with dignity.

Thus, it was said.

PREFACE

The fevers of Angola are of the same nature as those I have observed in other countries located in the Torrid Zone.[2] I have observed them in Rio de Janeiro, Bahia, and Pernambuco, though less frequently in these last two. The paroxysms, the crises, the progress, and the symptoms are all the same, and for this the methods of curing them that I am about to describe must be the same as those applied to fevers in other climates. I began to put them into action while in Rio de Janeiro, and the successes I then achieved convinced me to continue them in Angola, where I discovered a completely different treatment.

However, the opinion the Angolans have of doctors, which has been current in the country for many years, and the faith they maintain in the need for bloodletting in attacks of fever, have made them obstinate, which has in some measure hindered my efforts. I would have been of little use to the public had I not been employed as Physician General of that kingdom, which gave me complete jurisdiction over patients in the hospital. Little by little, if the people were convinced that the methods I followed were preferable, it is because they have seen that these techniques could save many people who, until then, they had never witnessed being cured under similar circumstances.

The abuse of bloodletting (which is still extraordinary in the cities of America, and especially in Salvador de Bahia) ended in Angola as the older physicians died; and with the instruction of new students, whom I trained by order of Your Majesty; and mainly as a consequence of the great difference in the number of deaths that occurred during my tenure, as compared to that of previous times. I do not claim to attribute this difference to my knowledge or to my talents, but rather to the progress medicine has lately made in the hands of other physicians from whom I have learned. It could not be expected that only medicine would remain in its backward state through the continuation of this illuminated and industrious age in which all other arts and sciences are being perfected. Since it is the greatest and most profound of the sciences, it has involved the greatest minds in its development; and in such proportion as its mysteries are revealed, it evidently will also discover new wonders.

After I had learned the general rules of medicine and its theories at university, I did nothing more than give voice to nature and observe when I was obliged to begin putting into practice the means of treating illness. Thus, my work is not the fruit of my imagination; rather, it is the result of my experience. The work I present to you is only my observations, both of the nature of the illnesses and of the means of treating them, because I do not seek to inflate the volume to produce a monstrous recompilation of all the writings there have ever been on this subject. I know that had I attempted to produce such a work it would prove useless, especially with an audience that has been served with the instructions of Pringle,[3] Lind,[4] Cleghorn,[5] Badenoch,[6] Clark,[7] Blane,[8] Hunter,[9] and many other erudite men.

In my experience with medical complaints, I observed among their symptoms the prognoses of which I found to agree with that which Hippocrates said in some of his *Aphorisms*; and therefore I have accentuated them, in honor of the father of medicine. It is true that when I treat the proximate cause of complaints I analyze the theories, hypotheses, and systems that are more prevalent on the matter, because the philosophizing mind belongs to he who seeks the truth, he who values experience, he who makes discoveries, and he who moves beyond empiricism. Far from being a satirist, I contradicted and opposed many opinions because I am permitted to think freely, because I love the truth and adore its image. However, I am sure my discourse contains many lapses and errors and that my conclusions do not always derive from the principles I state. Naturally, the spirit of man is not perfect and is easily inclined to express assumptions. However, I quickly alter my opinion and make immediate retraction when I notice an error and my mistakes are pointed out.

In the treatment of illnesses I state only the beneficial effects of the remedies of which I made use, and which I have found to be the most effective. I have also made use of many others cited as useful by authors, but as I have not shared the success they had, I do not speak of them here, thereby avoiding distracting the readers' attention. I was not as successful in the treatment of dysenteries as I was with fevers, despite making the greatest effort possible. Sydenham's treatments almost always failed,[10] Pringle's observations were few, and Hunter's attempts are yet to be judged. The damage dysentery causes in Angola is horrific, and its attacks dreaded because they are reputed to be totally incurable. I found that the medical authorities assumed the patient to be forsaken, and believed their skills useless and their art weak whenever the illness resisted their treatments for some days. I disavowed this inhumane abuse and set about trying to save many through my own diligence and devotion. Nonetheless, I confess my method of treating dysentery is as yet very imperfect. Future experiments and observations will perhaps have more favorable results than those we have experienced until now.

In no African illness did I work with so little success for so long as with tetanus, and in no other did I succeed in discovering a treatment as certain. My treatment has been put into practice by other physicians, who have attested to its efficacy and speed. My students have confirmed no more patients have died of tetanus after they had been shown the method of treatment. The antidotes are not new remedies: they are mercury and opium; what is new are the elevated doses that I found necessary to effect a cure. We are convinced that the ease with which we can now cure these intermittent fever outbreaks is a result of the large quantities of cinchona [quinine; "Peruvian bark"] that we administer to the patients, because the doses applied before did not have the same results and advantages that we have achieved.

Despite the continual work given me by patients in the hospital and the city, despite the effective diligence I require in order to continue the medical lectures with which I am charged and which use a great part of my time, on this occasion I would have written some other small essays from my jottings had the country's infirmities not haunted me so. Because my goal is to narrate facts and analyze phenomenon in order to decide the best method of treating diseases, which is the doctor's obligation, what I present here is neither ostentatiously eloquent nor of sublime style. I will be content if my labors have some use. My hopes will be fulfilled if this book is favorably received by the public.

Essay on the Fevers of Angola

Following Cullen,* I define fever as idiopathic pyrexia; that is, pyrexia without topical affection,[11] be it either essential or primary.†

This definition is essential for an understanding of primary fevers, which completely differ both in respect of their proximate and remote causes and in their treatment, which are symptomatic and a consequence of topical disorders, as is the case with exanthemas, discharges, hemorrhages, and *phlegmasia*.[12]

The *pyrexia*[13] resulting from topical affections is not a primary complaint, but rather is a symptom of the affection, and is therefore not a fever. There are no inflammatory fevers, because all inflammation causes local affection, of which the pyrexia is a symptom. If there is no topical blemish in the pyrexia, even though the pulse is strong and regular, the face flushed and red and without inflammation, this is because these symptoms do not always indicate it, nor are they enough to decide on the nature of the *phlogistic diathesis*.[14] The *synochus*[15] either did not exist or it was never *idiopathic*.[16] The general inflammation of the blood mass is hypothetical and without any foundation whatsoever.

Fever rarely consists of a single paroxysm. If there is some time between the end of one paroxysm and the beginning of another, during which there are no signs of fever, then this time is called the *intermission* and the fever *intermittent*. However, if instead of an intermission the fever only abates, then this relief is called *remission* and the fever is said to be *remittent*. If the patient and doctor are unaware of any

---

*William Cullen (1710–90), Scottish physician and leading figure in the Scottish Enlightenment. Cullen's *Synopsis nosologiae methodicae*, 2 vols. (Edinburgh, 1769; republished 1771, 1780, 1785), was a very influential "nosology," or systematic classification of diseases. It is hereafter referred to simply as Cullen's *Nosology*.—Trans.

José Pinto de Azeredo studied under Cullen's supervision at the University of Edinburgh. See William Cullen, *Works* (1827), vol. 1, p. 480.—Ed.

†See William Cullen, *Nosology* (1780), vol. 2, p. 43.

remission and the paroxysms appear labored and are continuous and unchanging, then the fever is called *continuous*.

All fevers have periods when their severity abates, even if only brief or unobserved. Thus we can say that, with the exception of symptomatic pyrexias, there are no fevers that can truly be called continuous. Therefore all fevers are either intermittent or remittent.

The old physicians, and even some modern ones, have introduced so many different kinds of continuous fevers that the study of them is tiresome and almost incomprehensible. There just needs to be one more symptom, or the fever just needs to be more serious, for them to create a new type of fever, even when both its cause and its treatment are the same. Thus, in order of the symptoms' severity, they have created a whole range of fevers: Amatoria, Amphimerina, Elodes, Lyngodes, Icterica, Ephemeral, Pemphigus, Putrid, Siriasis, Malignant, Burning, Judicatorial, Pemphygodes, Slow, Simple Continued, Encephalitis, Leipyria, Fricodes, Pernicious, Nervous, Bilious, etc.[17] This multiplication is entirely useless in practice and only serves to raise doubts and form hypotheses concerning the nature and cause of the same fever. In all fevers the treatment is practically the same: for all, if one seeks to treat just the symptom that is most serious, then, by that means only, it is sufficient to augment the primary complaint and impede it by removing its proximate cause. This is the problem the physician must always have in his mind to resolve. Laborious and confident observation is the only way to learn how to seek the methods most suitable for the treatment of the illness, and from those particular facts we will, like Bacon,[18] assess the general effects of the proximate cause and decide on the treatment to be administered in order to obtain a cure.

History of Remittent Fevers

All people, regardless of age and gender, can be attacked by remittent fevers, although men are struck more frequently than women, and adolescents more frequently than children. Perhaps this is so because men and adolescents have more exposure to the remote causes. It is certain that new arrivals to the African coast are attacked in greater force and with greater danger because they are unaware of the dangers of the sun and of the other causes and because of the habits they bring from more benign climates.

The ordinary manner[19] in which remittent fevers show is mainly through languor; inactivity; headache; tiredness; pains in the loins, joints, and bones; lack of appetite; a bitter taste in the mouth; nausea; chills in the back; rapid and irregular pulse; and bilious vomiting.

Sometimes all the symptoms appear together, at other times they appear separately and gradually increase, and the fever appears with the constant increase of heat in the body. When it is at its peak the pulse will increase and get stronger, harder, and more frequent; the throat and mouth become dry and the patient will have a continuous and un-quenchable thirst; anxiety increases, causing uneasiness and a tighten-ing in the chest; it turns the tongue white, [and] in the mouth secretions stop and breathing becomes labored.

It is not difficult to know whether the labored breathing is an effect of the fever or if it is caused by some topical disorder of the lungs. I have observed that labored breathing caused by a lung disorder is always uniform and that it is irregular when caused by fever. The patient takes three, four, or more normal breaths before breathing becomes labored and difficult again, which is how it continues for the duration of the paroxysm.

After some time all the symptoms diminish, the patient becomes sluggish, and the fever goes into remission. However, this is very ir-regular. Sometimes there is a great deal of perspiration, while at others there is only a slight dampness on the body or on the forehead, with the pulse remaining fast, the skin hot, and the face flushed.*

If the physician does not take immediate advantage of the remission by applying competent remedies, or, as is normally the case, the patient does not immediately contact the doctor, preferring instead to place his trust in nature, a second and much more dangerous and malignant paroxysm will befall him. This commonly presents itself with the re-

---

*Febricitanti sudor superveniens, febre non deficiente, malum [When the feverous person is overcome by sweat without the fever breaking, it is a bad sign—Trans.] [See Hippocrates et al., Hippocratis Aphorismi, Hippocratis et Celsi locis parallelis il-lustrati, studio et curâ Janssonii ab Almeloveen, D.M. . . . (Paris: Theophilum Barrois juniorem, 1784), 56:4. Azeredo is most likely to have used this edition.—Ed.]

turn of coldness in the back, or, even without any indication of this, the pulse will increase with such force it will be clearly visible in the carotid artery in the throat, the mouth will feel dry and rough like sandpaper, the tongue will be covered in a thick black coating that extends to the teeth,* the senses will be troubled and the mind confused, there will be memory loss, and finally delirium will be exhibited.

While remission from the first fit of fever is slight, the second is much less perfect. Relief from the symptoms of the exacerbated fit is only slight. While slowing, the pulse continues with the same strength. The skin dries and the patient feels great weakness. A short time later the fever will slowly increase and the patient will fall into a deep lethargy. Within a few hours patient will confuse his words; his senses will be affected and he will fall into an apoplectic and unconscious state.

Upon arriving at this unfortunate point, the fever will continue to rise without letting up in its violence. The patient's color will fade and take on a pallid cadaverous hue, the eyes will lose their shine and remain moribund and half closed, the pupils will dilate and will not react to rays of light, the mouth will remain half open, the muscles will be incapable of contracting, the hands will push constantly at the sheets or swat imaginary flies from the face. The entire body will be covered in a slow sweat, breathing will be fast and shallow, a constant low moan will accompany the difficult movement of the lungs until the moment finally arrives when the fit of fever normally remits and the poor unfortunate soul expires.†

Fevers do not always strike with the regularity described here. I have also seen that even when patients are delirious, their eyes remain wide open and they speak in a trembling and faltering voice that is not in their natural tone. Their chin trembles and they find it difficult to put their tongue out when required by the physician. If a question is asked, the patient will seek to respond, but will be unable to complete even a

---

Quibus in febre ad dentes viscosa circumnascuntur, his febres fiunt vehementiores. [When fevers are accompanied by a viscosity around the teeth, these fevers will strengthen.—Trans.] [See Hippocrates et al., *Hippocratis Aphorismi*, 53:4.—Ed.]

†*Ubi in febre non intermittente difficultas expirandi, e delirium fit, lethale.* [When, in a non-intermittent fever, dyspnea and delirium occur, the case is lethal.—Trans.] [*Hippocratis Aphorismi*, 50:4.—Ed.]

single word. In their imagination they are involved in important business requiring their activity, or they will invent hideous objects from which they wish to flee. They wish constantly to get out of bed, but as soon as they raise their head they will hold themselves in their arms and their entire body will begin to shake and they will fall back onto the bed should no one come to their aid. Thus such patients continue restless and afflicted, tossing from one side to the other without finding comfort until their strength is exhausted; they lose consciousness and collapse into a deep lethargy. At this point they experience shocks and convulsions in their tendons, they grind their teeth and begin to chew as if eating. It is while they are in this condition that they will die.*

However, while such patients' strength is not completely exhausted they will get out of bed in their delirium and wander through the house or hospital, either dressed or in their bedclothes, hurl themself at any precipice and not recognize anyone; the pulse can be only barely perceived, then it abruptly stops without any change of symptom.

Some patients fall into a lethargy without first experiencing delirium, and when they awaken they open their eyes, answer questions put to them, and immediately fall back into the same lethargy. They cannot explain their feelings or their first attack, and they look around them with an air of indifference, sighing often.

Although delirium is one of the symptoms that indicates the seriousness of the fever, it is not an essential ingredient, because patients are often very violent and malignant without either delirium or lethargy. In this way many fevers end in death when least expected. However, these fevers that prove fatal always have a moment in which they are in complete remission. Because of this the physician needs to have a precise understanding of what is a beneficial abatement and what is mortal in order to remind the patient of the steps that need to be taken. This

---

*In febre non intermittente, si labium, aut supercilium, aut oculus, aut nasus pervertatur, si non videat, si non audiat, corpore iam debili existente, quidquid horum fiat, in propinquo mors est. [In a non-intermittent fever, if the lip, the eyebrow, the eye, or the nose becomes contorted, if the patient neither sees nor hears, and the body is feeble—any one of these signs being present, death is near.—Trans.] [Hippocratis Aphorismi, 49:4.—Ed.]

knowledge is better obtained by practice than by description. However, I have included a short account of what experience has taught me.

If, after having made its remission, the fever leaves the skin cold and naturally moist, the pulse normal, the senses perfect and clear, it still leaves the patient extremely weak in body and spirit, with breathing that is tired, weak, and barely perceptible, drowsy and without appetite, having difficulty swallowing even his own saliva, with a complete aversion to the movement of any part of his body, while still tossing in bed from one side to the other, with a shallow and slow pulse, with cold extremities, and covered in perspiration at the same time that the patient says he is feeling well and in no discomfort, it is always certain that death is close at hand.* The pulse, which for all this time has been slow, will speed up during the final minutes, and the unfortunate patient will often be aware that death is close at hand through a feeling of weakness that greatly afflicts him. This, sadly, is how many fevers end, when the patient has suffered two or three violent attacks, even though none of the symptoms suggest any evident danger.

There are remittent fevers that are pernicious despite their symptoms seeming benign and requiring no care. These I describe here so that the physician can be forewarned and ready to administer the correct treatment in similar cases. In this type of fever the pulse is frequent but regular and beats with its natural strength, the soul functions perfectly without the slightest sign of delirium, the reaction is slight but does not diminish, and the skin temperature is natural and often totally fresh. However, the patient's face will be inflamed and his eyes red. Such patients will feel very hot inside, and they will experience tightness across their chest, they will toss and turn in bed and be unable to cool down, and no water will satisfy their thirst. Their mouth will be dry and their tongue inflamed.† This fever can last six, seven, or more days,

---

In morbis acutis extremarum partium frigus malum. [In acute maladies, the chilling of the extremities is bad. —Trans.] [*Hippocratis Aphorismi*, 1:7. —Ed.]

†*In non intermittentibus febribus, si externa quidem frigida sint, interna vero urantur, et sitim habeant, lethale.* [In a non-intermittent fever, if the external parts of the body are cold and the internal ones are burning, it is lethal. —Trans.] [*Hippocratis Aphorismi*, 48:4. —Ed.]

until the extremities get cold. The pulse is undetectable, but the patient is always in his right mind; however, the thirst will be more desperate and unquenchable. The patient persists with no perceptible pulse, and the body will get cold to the touch. Within the space of five hours, more or less, without giving any sign of impending death, the patient will suddenly take his last breath.

In some remittent fevers patients suffer from syncope [fainting] whenever they sit up in bed to eat soup or take some medicine, or for any other reason. Syncope is a sign the fever is mortal. I have witnessed this more normally in those who were copiously bled at the beginning of the attack of fever.

Fever is often accompanied with vomiting, which can be so violent that no treatment or food can be held in the stomach, with the patient eventually bringing up green bile and even blood, producing *black vomit*. The patient is at his weakest, and the fever, having taken control of the body, reaches its peak. After some days the vomiting, which has not responded to treatment, stops by itself and a mortal lethargy overcomes the patient's senses, which can only very rarely be restored.*

Jaundice appears in many remittent fevers, and is visible in the patient's eyes, urine, and over the entire skin. This symptom has given occasion for some authors to create a new class of fevers, which they call yellow, believing this color is caused by the dissolution of blood. I have not yet come across similar dissolution, and reason persuades me that the yellowing of the skin is a mere symptom; that is to say, it is the same jaundice caused and complicated by the fever.

In jaundiced fevers the eyes normally begin to show yellow at the end of the second or third paroxysm. The mortality that is often a result of these fevers is not the result of jaundice. I will not seek to explain why this symptom normally appears in those more dangerous fevers, for here I am a mere observer and chronicler of facts who must not offer opinions and conjecture.

---

*Morbis quibusvis incipientibus, si bilis atra, vel sursum, vel deorsum prodierit, lethale. [If at the commencement of any infirmity one evacuates black bile, whether vomited or excreted, it is a fatal sign.—Trans.] [Hippocratis Aphorismi, 22:4.—Ed.]

Should the patient survive the third and fourth paroxysms, and emerge free of fever, he will suffer other ailments no less consequential than this fever; because, finding the patient already weakened, the treatments become ineffectual, and thus any new ailments will become lethal. Dysentery is one of those that, commencing after a fever subsides, is rarely overcome.

Dysentery often occurs before fever, and often accompanies the fever, sometimes appearing in the midst of the fever and sometimes at the end. This complication never fails to be dangerous, particularly when it follows a fever; it is always to be taken seriously and requires the physician to pay it a great deal of attention and to apply all of his knowledge.

Convalescents are frequently subject to relapse, which is more dangerous than the first attack. The normal relapses are intermittent fevers that display no regularity in their frequency. From intermittent they become remittent, which are difficult to treat, and even if a cure is found, the patient will remain pale, thin, and cachectic.[20]

Attention must be paid to the liver during remittent fevers, because with the slightest fever this organ can become inflamed and blocked. If the inflammation is not treated quickly the organ will begin to suppurate, which will inevitably result in death. Hepatitis stimulated by fever is normally chronic, and because of the slightness of its symptoms is often neglected both by the patient and by some physicians who do not guard against the consequences and will address a similar complaint. As soon as the patient begins to feel pain on the part being palpated, no matter how slightly, and as soon as his breathing becomes labored after the fever has reached its peak, we must assume the liver is inflamed and obstructed.

In addition to the liver, the spleen is also prone to obstruction. This organ often grows in such a way that it occupies almost the entire abdominal cavity; however, inflammation of the spleen is very rare, and it never suppurates.

The obstruction of either of these organs often results in dropsy,[21] perhaps as a result of the compression of the trunks of the lymphatic vessels passing through them. Obstructions and dropsy can appear simultaneously without the latter being caused by the former. We have seen patients with edema at the end of some fevers when there is no suggestion of obstruction, just as we have seen obstructions that do not result in edema. Fevers, being often repeated, induce *cachexia*[22] throughout the system, particularly in the lymphatic vessels. Without being able to absorb the fluids deposited in the cavities they remain inert and allow the fluid to accumulate. In this way edema and obstruction can exist simultaneously without the former having been caused by the compression of the absorbent vessels. This distinction is essential for determining a treatment, because one form of edema requires treatment to remove obstructions, while the other requires stimulants and tonics.

When the obstructions become persistent, the attacks of fever will be accompanied by indigestion, flatulence, bilious vomiting, anxiety, and lack of appetite, which can be deduced from the changes in the obstruction. These small fevers are met with such indifference by those suffering from them that they ignore them, go outside and continue with their daily tasks without showing any outward concern about their fever. At other times those suffering may feel some languor, with slight headaches and with a bitter taste in their mouth, which they do not associate with symptoms of fever, when a fever is in fact what they have.

Remittent fevers also normally result in inflammation of the parotid glands, which will almost always suppurate.* With parotid inflammation, the termination of the fever is always dangerous. Because the patient's strength has been spent fighting the fever, the normal remedies for bringing down the inflammation are the very treatments that will increase the body's overall debility. Should these remedies be applied in order to prevent the very real danger of suffocation, the debility will increase and dysentery will result, from which there is little prospect of survival.

Should nature on occasion resist the fatal termination of parotid gland fever—because, even when the inflammation suppurates, this transpires over a long period of time—then it is important for the physician to know how to support the patient's rapidly diminishing

---

Lassatis per febres, ad articulos, et circa maxillas maxime absessus fiunt. [To those who experience languor during fevers, deposits form in the articulated joints, particularly next to the jaws. —Trans.] [*Hippocratis Aphorismi*, 31:4. —Ed.]

strength, which, failing every minute, provokes the dysentery of which we spoke above.

At the height of a fever I have witnessed the appearance of abscesses on various parts of the body, particularly in the anus; however, these are not dangerous and their suppuration comes easily, so that little or no intervention is required.

Following the end of the fever it is very common for patients to be left deaf and with an unpleasant ringing in their ears. They are often unable to smell, taste, or feel; however, all these signs are good. Following some crises of fever the limbs are paralyzed; however, this paralysis lasts at most two weeks before gradually wearing off. It is also very common for the patient to be stricken with scabs which appear on the body after the fever has gone, and which are commonly attributed to the use of warm remedies, particularly Peruvian bark,[23] although experience has convinced me they are nothing other than side effects of the fever.

In children remittent fevers are often accompanied with convulsions, as happens with smallpox. This has led some physicians to believe that the fevers are caused by stomach worms, and as they seek to expel them they increase the fever, which remains untreated and thus only makes matters worse.

Another symptom that appears on rare occasions is the effusion of water on the ventricles of the brain. I have seen this twice in children. I attended an examination to observe all of the symptoms of hydrocephalus in some children with fevers, and I discovered the cause in the dissections. However, I have never seen these effusions in adults.

Remittent fevers can also lead to tetanus or lockjaw, which are always fatal in these cases.

In some, at the end of five or six days I have seen open sores on all those parts of the body that are compressed with the weight of the body in its normal posture, such as the buttocks, the parts around the greater trochanter, and the spine of the ileum. Having no connection whatsoever with the fever, it is a very bad sign, and few if any patients survive it. These sores are proof the life force is very fragile, and that parts of the body can be destroyed because they have lost their tone.

Tremors in the hands are another very common and unfortunate symptom. This will increase in proportion to the weakening of the pulse, and as delirium increases; this will continue during the abatement of the illness. The tremors indicate an increased debility induced by the fever in the body's moving fibers, combined with the threat of subsequent increased bouts of fever.

In other fevers pale livid spots appear below the surface of the skin. These eruptions are confluent, attacking arms, legs, backs, chests, and occasionally the face. These *petechiae*[24] I cannot consider critical, because they are as likely to appear during those fevers that are merely dangerous as they are in those that are fatal and in those fevers that simply vanish. In all, the fevers in which they are discovered must be treated with care and attention. I have even seen them appear some hours after the death of a fever patient.

It is necessary to be cautious and not to confuse these petechiae with those that are the consequence of the scurvy that often complicates the fever, especially on the coast of Africa. It is not difficult to distinguish whether these are a symptom of the fever or scorbutic diathesis within the system. Scorbutic petechiae are not normally regular in size and are black, small or large, and appear across the entire body. Fever petechiae are always very small and pale. Scorbutic petechiae are accompanied with lacerated gums and loose teeth, while fever petechiae begin to appear after the third febrile peak. Attention must be paid to this distinction in order to ascertain which of the completely different treatments is appropriate.

Urine also changes with fever. As the fever rises the urine becomes as red as blood; however, as the time of crisis peaks,[25] the urine becomes richer and contains sediment. I have seen murky, pale, clear, and transparent urine as the fever is at its peak. Given that the changes are irregular, there is no prognosis to help the physician in his examination. I eventually disregarded them, despite the authority of so many physicians who, with Hippocrates, confirmed the need for a similar examination.*

---

*Per vesicam prodeuntia inspicere oportet, an sint qualia sanis prodeunt. Quae igitur minime his similia, ea morbosiora; sanis vero similia, minime morbosa. [One needs to verify that the patient's gallbladder secretions are the same in sickness as in health. When they are dissimilar, they are bad; similar secretions are not diseased.—Trans.] [Hippocratis Aphorismi, 66:7.—Ed.]

One of the outcomes I believe to be favorable is hemorrhage, especially from the nose, from which the blood does not coagulate. It also commonly happens that the patients' lips, mouth, and tongue split open, all of which can be considered to provide an optimistic prognosis.

Physicians who closely and blindly observe the doctrines of Hippocrates even today await the fever's critical days. Some of those writing this century are merely repeating ancient doctrines rather than reflecting on them, and allow their inviolate respect for the opinions [of these doctrines] to pass into our days. Even Cullen, my wise master, being a free and eclectic man, fell into the same error concerning the critical days. Cullen followed the Hippocratic doctrine of similar days, using as proof the periodic movements observed continually among all animals, both when healthy and when sick.*

However, the very movements observed in the healthy state by Cullen are visible results of physical causes that also operate for periods of time. The very movements observed among illnesses are not the result of the curative force of nature discovered by Stahl,† and supported by Cullen,‡ but rather they are the result of other causes described in their place.§ I have witnessed fevers end both on the so-called critical days as well as on noncritical days. Cullen's claim, therefore, is improbable. Accepting the idea of critical days means the physician, waiting for the crisis, stops providing the treatment that is necessary at that time, when it is most necessary, which will perhaps cost the patient his life. We can admit critical days, but only as long as they are not used to hinder the continuation of necessary treatment.

We are now convinced Stahl's system is entirely hypothetical.

---

*See William Cullen, *First Lines of the Practice of Physic*, §§ 107–24. [See John Thomson, ed., *Works of William Cullen, M.D ... Containing His Physiology, Nosology and First Lines of the Practice of Physic ...* , 2 vols. (Edinburgh and London: William Blackwood and T. & G. Underwood, 1827), vol. 1, pp. 591–98.—Ed.]

†See Stahl, *Theoria medica vera*. [Georg Ernst Stahl (1659–1734), German physician who wrote *Theoria medica vera: Physiologiam et pathologiam. . . .* (Halle: Typis et Impensis Orphanotrophei, 1706–8).—Ed.]

‡See Cullen, *First Lines of the Practice of Physic*, vol. 1, pp. 38–39. [See also Cullen, *Works* (1827), vol. 1, p. 493.—Ed.]

§See *Causa proxima*, pp. 34–35. [This note refers to the original page numbers of the 1799 publication; now pp. 80–81, below.—Ed.]

Proximate Cause

Up to now I have not departed from a narration of facts and have sought to avoid all conjecture and speculation. I have merely recounted with care and caution the observations made during my study.

However, seeking to investigate the proximate cause of fevers in order to discover a method of cure that is scientific rather than empirical, I find myself obliged to discourse metaphysically and to draw inferences that serve as generic notions for this same end. Although many argue theories are of no use, I find myself unable to separate them from practice. It is not enough for us to have knowledge of palpable things; our senses are few and imperfect and are of little use unless they are guided by reason, which is more sublime. Physics furnishes us with solid principles from which we take abstract conclusions, and these consequences serve as generic rules that are also new principles in which we discover other physical truths of which our senses are unaware. Thus they are mutually given into our hands and must always remain inseparable. There will never be progress if we use one without the other. In this way I proceed to study opinions on the nature and cause of fevers, following which I will narrate some of my views.

I have no wish to recount the systems that appeared in the early years of medicine as a way of combatting the erroneous opinions of these dark centuries. It is tiresome to seek to convince and persuade those who are convinced and persuaded otherwise. Asclepiades's ideas,[26] though they were carried forward in the method announced by Themison,[27] in which the empirical sect was destroyed, does not have the glory to persist. Despite Celsus's eloquence,[28] his ideas fade with the appearance of Galen[29] and the new medical system, which seems to be more correct. All the qualities Galen supposed to be the cause of diseases were discredited through the proofs presented by Paracelsus and his school.[30] However, the chemical pathology that flowered then began to be neglected to the extent that, through dissections, the anatomical school began discovering new functions in the human body. The innate primal heat and radical moisture was reputed to be an imaginary cause when Harvey, discovering the circulation of the blood, thought the fever was caused by the disordered movement of the blood through the excessive exaltation of the spirits.[31]

However, Sydenham, the most astute observer of nature, who, like Bacon, had learned to despise vain conjectures and to gather facts, set about describing illnesses to physicians who had only paid attention to the explanation of ether. In this way the theories of that time were destroyed, and there were discovered copious cures for a thousand ill-nesses that had been attributed to very different causes. It was enough for Baglivi to prove the action of moving fibers as the engines of the animated body,[32] for physicians to return their attention to the move-ment of solids and to stop believing in the existence of a viscous fluid, or *lentor*,[33] within the extremities of the small vessels in which the fever originates. Persuaded of this truth, they ceased seeking to expel the lentor, because it is known that medication works as a stimulant that affects the common sensory function through the movement of nerves.

When curing fevers, Pitcairn[34] sought to encourage secretions from the natural passages, or *meatus*, of the skin, which had been hindered and complicated by the acrimony of the nervous fluid. Further, suppos-ing this to be an impediment to the fevers' immediate cause, the proof of which was the success of his practice, he prompted the abandonment of all opinions that had prevailed in this respect up to his day. A selec-tion of some of Borelli's[35] mechanical principles and Lemery's chemical principles constitute a system that attacks Pitcairn's pathology.[36]

Boerhaave,[37] a physician of vast erudition, could destroy all his pre-decessors' systems, bringing to the fore a new pathology. The acrimony of the fluids and the pathogenic, or *morbific*, materials taken or gener-ated within the blood's mass emerges as the cause of many illnesses. Fevers are already produced by too much bile in the stomach and by its fermentation. Pringle argued there is a strong tendency toward rot in the blood and the humors, and it is this that causes the fever. In all, both systems are weakened when, through means of a perfect analysis of blood, Hewson seeks to convince us that the blood within the vessels is always pure.[38]

The authority of these schools is further diminished by the lessons of Cullen, who, in agreement with what Hoffman[39] said about moving fibers, and convinced by Haller's experiments,[40] by Whytt's[41] observations, and by Gaubius's principles,[42] created a new doctrine that sought to destroy the maxims of the humorists. They revived Willis's[43] long-dead ideas as Cullen acquired the name of the creator and father of modern medicine. The origin and proximate cause of the complaints were sought in the nerves, which are the living solids and the only organs of our sensations and of our functions. A spasm formed in the moving fibers of the extreme vessels, particularly those at the surface of the skin, thus comes to be the proximate cause of fevers in general.

Cullen's doctrine seems to me to be closest to the truth, and being approved in practice by its successes has gained credit and flourishes. Although a certain doctor Brown appeared, intent on destroying Cullen's system with a theory that is entirely the product of a fertile imagination,[44] Brown's theory has withered of itself and has demonstrated its insufficiency in practice. While Brown's principles correspond to some facts of nature, they are not enough to form a general system of medicine. The oversimplicity of Brown's principles led reckless physicians into making fatal errors and held the prudent in continual confusion and indecision. The proximate cause of fevers as explained by Brown is not new, only the name he gave it was. What Brown called asthenia, Cullen called weakness or atony.

I am convinced there are spasms upon the surface of the body in all fevers, whether they be inflammatory or nervous. Once the moving fibers are disturbed and lose their natural state, as a general rule of the natural economy of animals,[45] they have a propensity to spasm.

However, with the debility and the consequent spasm being the proximate cause of nervous fevers, how can the fever cease for some time (the intermission) and then lead to another paroxysm if its cause still exists within the system? How can this cause, which has not left the body, permit the fever to fade for some hours, or even days?

A short consideration is enough to find the response to this objection. All causes always need the disposition of nature, and because of this they do not always function. The intermission is not a result of the debility that caused the fever, but rather it is an effect of the paroxysm that managed to remove the spasm. The opium administered in many cases relieves many pains, and this relief persists for as long as the effects of the opium last; however, as soon as it wears off, the pain and the other symptoms return, and often with greater force, because their causes were suppressed only by virtue of the remedy. The untimely administration of opium in cases of dysentery decreases evacuations and removes pains and tenesmus[46] for several hours, but as soon as its effect begins to wear off, all these symptoms appear with greater force for the simple reason that the treatment had not removed the cause of the illness. In the same way, in fevers the increased action of the heart and the arteries relaxes the spasms, and this relaxation is prolonged for the whole time that the debility is suppressed by the effect of increased action of the heart; and, as the intermission consists of the relaxation of the spasm, that thus continues until the debility is again able to renew the spasm. This way of explaining nature's actions seems to me to be closest to the truth, and completely undermines the "healing force of nature" that Cullen, without need, seeks to sustain.

Remote Causes

For me to enter into a particular examination of the remote causes of fevers and other maladies in Angola, I must occupy the readers' attention with a brief description of the country. Its land, its waters, its plants, its atmosphere, its winds, its customs, and its food perhaps offer the inquiring mind some interesting news through which it can discover the most effective ways of preventing and remedying so many ills. I am convinced that endemic illnesses depend on a single common cause that exists in the atmosphere and which is always hidden from us. History shows us that when struck by epidemics, it was more prudent for military generals to move their camps to a different location than to depend on the safeguards of the wisest physicians. Moreover, this general cause will not function without the necessary conditions[47] also existing. It is these I will now proceed to relate.

It is not recognition of the causes in general that plagues the life of man and that led me to describe those that in Angola seem to have been given the ability to lay low a numerous population, and which undermined its prior opulence; rather, it is through my zeal for the country in which I live and for the conservation of which I care so much.

The principal city of Angola is situated on land that is arid, sterile, dry, sandy, and strewn with loose gravel.[48] Because of the lack of bedrock, the annual rains change its appearance. It has no fresh water, so the people drink the water of the River Bengo that, because of the distance, is brought by sea in canoes. This water cannot but be anything but awful, since the riverbed is of mud, it has a current so slow moving as to be barely perceptible, and it is inhabited by huge alligators, or crocodiles, that seek only to make prey of any living thing that comes down to the riverbank. They graze on the countless numbers of unsuspecting people who go to take water. Rather than seeking to clean the water, the inhabitants of Bengo continually dump into it the spoils from their plantations: the dead leaves, rotting logs, and other unclean waste. This water, even when filtered through stones as it normally is, and even when perfectly clear, remains a vehicle for corrupting human flesh in which so many putrid substances ferment, and can never be pure and healthy. No matter how small the stones through which the water is filtered, they cannot separate the very small particles within it, those that are so small we cannot perceive them with our senses.

There is a well in Maianga (a place a short distance from Luanda) that supplies water to a large number of the people. No matter how much water is drawn, there is always a foot of water in this well: its level never rises or falls, but remains the same. However, this water is heavy and brackish, and it contains a lot of earth that is easily separated through evaporation. Soap will not easily dissolve in it. Its bad taste is attributed to its adulteration with water from the sea, which is very close to the well. I have sometimes noticed that this water tastes more unpleasant at high tides. The earth with which the water is combined seems to consist of gypsum components, which do not separate through the stone filters the inhabitants use to purify it.

In other times people used the water from the Island of Luanda, which is close to and opposite the city of Luanda, and the water from Missengle, a peninsula which with the island forms the Corimba Bank. Both places, which are made of sand and are unsuitable for agriculture, are inhabited only by fishermen. The way in which they collect water is remarkable. They dig a hole less than a foot deep, which fills in a minute with perhaps the best fresh water in all Angola. The people stopped making their small wells in these places because of the work and inconvenience involved, because whenever more water was needed it was necessary to dig a new hole, as after even one day the water in the existing holes would become salty. There is not a common opinion about the source and nature of this water, and many would like to believe the water is from the sea filtered through the sand, but I think this improbable given that water taken from holes close to the shoreline is equally fresh. I am of the opinion that below this land there is a tributary of the river Cuanza, or of another river, and that this is the true origin of this water.

On the beach at Cassandama, which is about a league from Luanda, there is a small and completely ignored source. Its water has a reputation for being harmful and for causing diarrhea. In my analysis of this water I found it contained much gypsum and sulfur, both of which are abundant in this area. It is a benign laxative that can be used daily; and as such on many occasions I have successfully applied it in some chronic complaints.

Educated people in the country drink the rainwater that is collected in a large cistern in the Fortress of São Miguel. Because of its cleanliness, this keeps the water pure and in the best possible condition.

As there is little rain in Angola, there are very few plants that grow without dependence on collected rainwater, and hardly any trees. Their usefulness to the population means there is an urgent public need for the conservation of cisterns, as well as for a planned increase in their number.

We must give credit to the recent experiments of Ingenhousz[49] and other modern philosophers who have shown that plants breath, and that by doing so they absorb *mephitic air*, or nitrogen,[50] from the atmosphere and replace it with oxygen. Therefore, it seems plants provide us with a large portion of the pure air that men use to breathe and to live. This is reason enough to prove the need for their existence in populated areas. I realize this especially when the air turns worse, such as that which is breathed in the pestilential region of Batavia after the government cut down the majority of the trees lining its streets. It is better that trees be broadly distributed because, rather than being useful, dense woods and forests are prejudicial to health, with their rotting leaves generating impure and noxious air, their canopies cutting off light, their density preventing air from circulating, and by providing a home for infinite animals that infest the atmosphere.

The majority of trees in Africa produce quantities of resins and fragrant balsams that, with their scent, correct the effects of corruption. However, they only emerge and grow in the distant hinterlands, which perhaps because of this are, like Benguela, healthier and more benign. Within Luanda and its environs the most commonly seen plants are those Angolans call *canuminumi*,[51] *massambala*,[52] *catolotólo*,[53] *muxixi, embondo*,[54] *zumzo, quitalango*,[55] *muxaxaquixe*,[56] *quibuma* (sweet basil), *mupondolo*,[57] *murianhoca*,[58] and others about which I have no knowledge. Many forms of jasmine grow in the country, and these are just as fragrant, if not more so, than those to be found in Europe.

Noting the uses and usefulness of trees for the colonists and natives of the colony, we ought to insist on their conservation, or even call for an increase in their numbers. Rather than purchase material, the poor natives make much use of the few remaining baobab trees to make fasteners of various kinds, with the twine as thread for their beads. The bark is used to cover the nudity of the industrious Quissama people and of the poor slaves who doubtless resist hunger and scurvy by eating the mealy pulp of the fruit that remains fresh within its double pod.[59]

The *muxixi*, the seeds of which provide nourishment for birds that provide the town with a courtly feast for the eyes with their color and a royal feast for the ears with their song, provides excellent materials, particularly for the coopers who use the rattan to create the frames for many of the casks they construct. The root of the young *muxixi* tastes like sweet cassava (the root plant that in the Americas is used to make flour for bread), and both it and its leaf shoots provide excellent sustenance.

In addition to its medicinal and economic values, the *cassoneira*, which is certainly a type of euphorbia, has a very white wood that serves to provide a cool shade protecting the tender grasses from the rays of the sun. The *catolotólo* is good firewood and provides dense shade, even being capable of eliciting curiosity in Europe, where it is made into delicate green-black boxwood objects. The *canuminúmi*,[60] *quibondo*,[61] *mupondolo, insandeiras*[62] trees and the rest are no less useful, providing firewood and sustenance for many poor people, helping the economy of the wealthy, and the roots of which secure loose and shallow soil.

The continual droughts prevent abundance in the country of these plants that man requires for the conservation of his health and his life and which prevent scurvy, that malady of Luanda that infects almost all its inhabitants and which provokes such lamentable wastage in the human species.[63] There are few who cultivate these plants owing to the difficulty in finding, possessing, and conserving them. Fruit is lower in quality but greater in abundance because the trees are better able to resist the heat of the sun. They are all capable of being good, particularly oranges, which are as good as those produced in Europe. This excellent fruit is the only one capable of preventing scurvy and of reversing its onset. The others serve more to delight the palate. The pineapple is the equal of, if not superior to, that of America, while the mango is perhaps the equal of that found in India.

Kola nut is a solid and bitter fruit of which the inhabitants make constant use, chewing it at all times with water, which it makes sweet and tasty, as is the case with almost all bitters. By being used for its qualities, it aids digestion, and because of these benefits it has become such a luxury that companions offer pieces of it, which they call "legs," to one another as a courtesy, with the same gallantry with which we exchange snuff between us.

Many are the causes that have by necessity made the climate pestilent, the most terrible of which is in my opinion the sun. Even the strongest and most robust man's mortality is evident whenever he is exposed to the sun for any length of time. The heat in the place in which one walks is enough to provoke a fever. Experience has shown me that those who stay out of the sun are those who remain fit and healthy. The soldier who because of his obligations cannot take precautions from the sun, the miserable exiled convict laborer, and the poor who do not have the means to sustain themselves and who beg on the streets, are those who suffer the insults of the country and who tend not to survive. The same officers who in Luanda enjoy perfect health soon fall ill when service obliges them to be exposed to the sun's rays. During campaigns and detachments, when the troops need to march in the heat of the day, fevers and dysenteries tend to cause more damage than the enemy's bullets.

Today, as a result of the providence of Your Majesty's governors, there are no swamps or pools of stagnant water in the vicinity of Luanda, but they are all some distance away. During the rainy season the water of the River Bengo breaks its banks and floods the surrounding countryside, with the water retained in the soil for several months thereafter. Physicians have always believed the gases given off by these waters to be poisonous to the human body. The ground that was submerged gives off a gas that is fatal when breathed without being mixed with fresh air.*

It is not easy to determine the distance the miasma from these pools can reach. Clark and Robertson claim it is less than two miles,† although it all depends on the size of the pool, the position and height of the hills, and the speed and direction of the wind.

The Bengo, which is about four leagues from Luanda, is a very unhealthy place, and it is very unusual for people to go there without returning seriously ill. While never good, it is less dangerous in winter, during the misty season, because the air has fewer noxious vapors given off by the rotting plants, even though the fields are free of surface water. Cannot the gases given off by some of these vast stagnant pools be carried on the winds to Luanda and poison the air there? And could this not be equally bad, were it not for its proximity to the sea?

It seldom rains in Angola, but it is during the rainy season that the level of illness increases, of a type that is commonly referred to as the *carneirada*.[64] I have noted that showers are more dangerous because they only draw up vapors from the ground, which are then heated by

---

*Vid. Phil. Trans. vol. 69, p. 337. [See Felix Fontana, "Experiments and Observations on the Inflammable Air Breathed by Various Animals. By the Abbe Fontana, . . . Communicated by John Paradise, Esq. F. R. S.," *Philosophical Transactions of the Royal Society of London* 69 (1 January 1779): pp. 337–61.—Ed.]

†Vid. Clark's Observations on Voyages to the East Indies. Vid. Robertson's Physical Journey kept on board of His Majesties ship. [See John Clark, *Observations on the Diseases in Long Voyages to Hot Countries: And Particularly on Those Which Prevail in the East Indies* (London: D. Wilson and G. Nicol, 1773); Robert Robertson, *A Physical Journal Kept on Board His Majesty's Ship* Rainbow, *during Three Voyages to the Coast of Africa and West Indies, in the Year 1772, 1773, and 1774. . . .* (London: E. and C. Dilly, 1777).—Ed.]

the sun to create a thick and pestilent air that is impossible to breathe. Heavy rains are not as damaging because they clear the air, precipitating the heterogeneous particles that flow or combine with it. There is a saying in Angola: "When it rains there is much food, but no one to eat it." It is true that at these times the illnesses and diets do not let one enjoy the land's new produce. The rains come but twice a year, and that is enough to fertilize the fields and ensure an abundance of vegetables.

In my experience, the most critical part of the year is the hot seasons: the months of March, April, and May are fearful and their attacks pernicious.

Mere humidity is not the culprit, or at least it is not capable of producing fever. However, when the humidity comes through the soles of the feet it often causes serious illnesses, and particularly fevers and dysenteries.

There are other accidental causes that compete with the impurity of the atmosphere. The immense number of slaves, which commerce brings from all parts of the wilderness to the center of Luanda, and even into the homes of businessmen, where they remain until an occasion arises to transport them to Brazil; the fish that for many days are left in the sun on the city's beaches after being gutted, always covered in flying insects, including flies and botflies, until the fish is dried; the large straw houses that the rains rot and cause to decay, leading them to release noxious gases;[65] the huge number of cadavers that lay poorly buried in ground incapable of consuming them in the cemeteries and churches: these are undoubtedly the causes of a thousand illnesses. Such must be valid matters for the cogitations, the studies, and the concern of those who are responsible for the public good. Nothing matters in the villages more than health. It is no less certain that this goal is being taken seriously everywhere by the magistrates who, thank goodness, keep watch on all circumstances that may lead to such a welcome end. While the causes mentioned may prove difficult to remove, it is not impossible to remove them. Diligence will always prevail when set against difficult obstacles.[66]

All these causes would be more active, the illnesses always fatal, and the land wholly uninhabitable should certain infallible winds cease to blow each day and cool the air, remove the stillness, introduce more pure gases, and remove any amount of effluvia damaging to human life. In the space of twenty-four hours these winds will blow from every point of the compass: in the morning they blow from the land, and in the afternoon they blow from the sea, always bringing freshness with them. Despite the intense heat the days are bearable for those who protect themselves from the sun's rays. The nights, which are always accompanied by a gentle zephyr, are agreeable; particularly those nights that are illuminated by the light of the moon, which can be so clear it almost seems to wish to compete with the sun. The higher part of the city, which is always washed over by breezes, is for this reason the healthiest, and therefore most suitable for habitation. Those who live on the beach, on the lower part, live where the air is more still, and suffer repeated illness, though they experienced a great difference for the better after they took down the wall of the raised walkway surrounding São Miguel that had been preventing the circulation of breezes.

The black people, however, live with the whites and learn their customs, observe their religion, and speak their language without ever forgetting their own rites, customs, and heathen superstitions. When they are ill they do not seek physicians, and neither do they take pharmaceutical remedies; they have faith only in their own medicines, which they call *milongos*, and which must be administered by witch doctors or folk healers. It is to be regretted that many whites born in Angola, and even some Europeans, have faith in the virtue of such remedies and covertly seek the assistance of similar healers. They seek to defend their superstitions and the error of their ways by noting that many cases of maladies that physicians consider incurable have been miraculously overcome by black traditional practitioners. However, many are the disgraces that happen every day in this medicine based on ignorance, abuse, and illusion! How many illnesses that are by nature benign become mortal when their treatment is entrusted to the hands of these charlatans? Without doubt in the rural backcountry, an infinite number of people die simply as a result of the barbarous methods with which they are treated. Some native heathens live for years with ingrained maladies they do not know how to cure, and which would respond to our remedies and soon be cured should they come to have the good fortune to be treated by trained true physicians.

The custom among the black people to mourn the dead through what they call *entambe* is the source of vices, excesses, irreligion, and illness. They do not respond to the preaching of priests or to the sword of the church; nor has the strength of the secular authorities been able to end these heathen ceremonies. Both sexes come together in the home of the dead and close the doors, and as soon as the body is taken to be buried they remain in the dark for several days, wailing all the time for the dead and loudly lamenting the dead person's loss to their children, parents, and friends. However, this deference done for the widow or widower, or whichever relative, is always accompanied with a great deal of wine, a great deal of *alo* (a drink they make from fermented corn), and a great deal of counterfeit Brazilian *aguardente* manufactured in local taverns, venereal excesses, and many other disorders, with disastrous consequences.

It has been the general consensus of physicians since the earliest times that the immoderate use of spirituous liquors encourages illnesses that are endemic to that climate which they inhabit. Experience has shown this proposition to be true, indeed so true that to deny it is a simple absurdity.

Hoffman said that spirituous liquors are the most unwholesome because they inflame the solids within the body, coagulate the bodily fluids, and cause obstructions in the viscera, leading to the hectic fevers and edemas that affect many citizens, destroying their stomachs, intestines, livers, and lungs. Nevertheless, despite the fact that this great physician wrote with such sincerity in favor of his compatriots, about their singular fatality, that simply tolerating their monstrous abuses seems only to perpetuate their regrettable mistakes.

The Lord Bishop of Worcester, full of love for humanity's well being, delivered a moving sermon in London in which he claimed the use of hard liquors was the main reason for the depopulation of England, that these liquors were the cause of all illnesses among the people, and that they were also the cause of all manner of crimes.[67] I believe it is useless to make so much effort to explain the progress and successive changes in our bodies' response to wine and liquor. The entire world is well aware of their effects. We clearly recognize that, in those we find inebriated, the mouth is always dry and the saliva thick, with the

appearance of egg whites, which proves the great change and altera-
tion in the saliva glands and in their excretory ducts. The crapulence
caused by alcohol affects the strength of the entire system, disturbs
the brain's function, diminishes nerve sensations, causes the moving
fibers to lose their strength, and prevents the solids from exercising
their functions. Similar transformations in bodies cannot but result in
most serious illnesses.

Venereal excesses are another cause of fevers. They take all the
strength, weaken the structure, deplete the blood of its balsam, use
up all energy, cause weight loss that leads even men of robust constitu-
tions, and who are capable of living for a century, to have short lives.
I am convinced that a single venereal act in Africa produces as much
debility as may be induced by a major surgical bloodletting. With that
fire, the basic principle of life, so essential, stifled, the nerves weaken,
the entrails become inactive, the harmony that relies on the action and
reaction of solids and fluids declines little by little, there is a loss of
equilibrium, and the relaxation of the organs does not allow the weight
of the machine to be supported. This general weakening brings fatal
disorders in its wake, the most frequent of which in every African country is fever.

In addition to these, there are other vices that also result in, or which
are at least responsible for, fevers. This is the case with the abuse of
large, heavy meals that lead to indigestions, when the weakened bowels
are incapable of supporting reckless gluttony; the continuous all-night
vigils that, as innocent as they are, disturb the body's functions by rob-
bing it of the sleep that sustains it; the lack of cleanliness, both of body
and of clothing, has a great influence on the rates of illness.

Poor diet also helps the progress of illness, further increasing the fee-
bleness of bodies already affected by the heat that keeps people slowly
and continually sweating. The best food, which is also the most con-
sumed, is fish; it is best not only because it is abundant and cheap, but
also because of its flavor. The beef, while scarce, is excellent, although
it is eaten most by Europeans. The bread favored by the indigenes is
made from yucca flour, which, while lighter than bread made from
wheat, has the virtue of being antiscorbutic. They use a lot of palm oil
in their dishes, which they eat with *infunge*, a large cake made from rice

or corn flour. Their sauces contain too much pepper, of which there are many species. The peanut, which in Brazil is called *amendoim*,[68] is very popular, and sustains a large proportion of the people, despite its being indigestible. There is also *quicoanga*, which is made from cassava kept under water to ferment, and which in Brazil is called *puba*, and which has a very pleasant taste. Children eat *matete*, which is a very moist porridge made of *fuba*—rice or corn flour—or from shredded *quicoanga*.

The blacks do not eat very much: a kola nut chewed with a cup of water is enough for lunch. Two cobs of corn will be enough to sustain a man who has to make a journey of several days. During the dry season they will eat insects such as locusts, and several other animals.

While all the causes mentioned here may or may not be the cause of illness in the country, I dare not address them and leave it to the judgment of the readers to decide.

Cure

I return once more to outlining my observations of the use of some remedies that to me seem useful for removing fevers. Placing to one side the opinions of some authors whose practices have been followed as being more certain and better, I refer only to my own sentiments. While I have always respected their authority, I have never had so much faith in them that I follow them blindly; I have always sought to be guided by reason and discourse. The cure for fevers I present here, the observations on the application of treatments, the experiences of their successful outcomes, are the result of my diligence and my research.

There is no illness that requires swift attention more than fever. The effectiveness of the remedies almost always depends on their prompt administration. The illness gains strength each time it is allowed to run its course, and waiting for it to reach its crisis is time lost, when it is not indeed fatal. The physician must not lose a moment, nor must he be indifferent to the smallest symptoms, because these quickly grow to become mortal. Close attention must be paid to everything, and everything must be taken seriously. Home remedies, such as those with which the patient is normally treated, have in these cases often been the cause of death.

Should I see a patient at the beginning of his attack of fever, during the first paroxysm, I will normally administer an antimony emetic right away.* As well as bringing up the bile in the bowels, this will cause strong diaphoresis (perspiration), which will reduce any fever that may still be increasing. The patient will feel some relief sometime after the administration of the emetic. Having achieved complete remission from fever, which will be evident by the sweat and the reduction of symptoms, this time should be used to give an eighth of Peruvian bark each hour until an ounce has been administered. This is sufficient to prevent a subsequent paroxysm. This simple and easy method ordinarily cures many fevers that, treated in other ways, prove fatal.

However, there are times when the fever does not respond to the emetic and when there is no reduction in its growth. In such cases I will always first try to reduce the agitation and reaction of the same fever by administering a good dose of opium combined with the same antimony in a dose sufficient to provoke nausea.† This treatment is the most forceful I have come across to secure remission, and it very rarely fails.

Feces retained in the intestines are often the reason for a fever continuing. The administration of an antiphlogistic purgative can loosen the bowels, making them more pliable and softening the stool, which can lead to remission. The more appropriate purgatives are neutral salts.‡ On occasions when the bowels appear more resistant I administer the purgative with some manna.§

---

*Tartarized antimony; two grains in hot water (two ounces); dissolve. [See *Pharmacopoeia Collegii Regalis Medicorum Londinensis* (London: Josephum Johnson, 1788), p. 53; and *Pharmacopeia Geral para o Reino e Domínios de Portugal*, 2 vols. (Lisbon: Regia Officina Typografica, 1794), vol. 2, p. 131. For pharmaceutical measurements see *Pharmacopoeia... Londinensis*, pp. 1–3, and *Pharmacopeia Geral*, vol. 1, pp. 7–9. —Ed.]

†Opium tincture, forty drops; antimony wine, thirty drops; simple cinnamon water, one ounce; stir. [See *Pharmacopoeia... Londinensis*, p. 100; *Pharmacopeia Geral*, vol. 2, p. 212.—Ed.]

‡Vitriolic soda or vitriolic magnesium, two ounces; hot water, six ounces; dissolve. [Neutral salts are balanced, neither acid nor alkaline. See *Pharmacopoeia... Londinensis*, p. 44; *Pharmacopeia Geral*, vol. 2, p. 174.—Ed.]

§Vitriolic soda or vitriolic magnesium, one and a half ounces; hot water, six ounces; dissolve. Manna, one and a half ounces; mix. [*Pharmacopoeia... Londinensis*, p. 44; *Pharmacopeia Geral*, vol. 2, p. 174.—Ed.]

If following the administration of the purgative the fever continues at the same level, then I replicate the dose with a second drink of opium with antimony, which almost never fails to produce the desired result.

As soon as the remission begins, I waste no time in administering one and a half ounces of Peruvian bark in two-eighths doses each hour. There are certainly some stomachs that cannot tolerate such doses of pure undiluted Peruvian bark. In these cases I will reduce the dose, but never to less than one-sixteenth every hour. However, there are stomachs yet that cannot even accept such a small dose, where I have had to boil the Peruvian bark and administer it in an infusion in three-ounce doses every two hours.* Using a decoction or an infusion of the bark is often much more useful than in those cases in which the Peruvian bark is administered in its pure form, perhaps because it reaches the stomach's nerves more quickly. However, whenever possible it is preferable to introduce the pure Peruvian bark, undiluted.

I have frequently used *água de Inglaterra*,[69] which is worth the effort in difficult cases; however, I have never thought it to be more effective than powdered Peruvian bark; rather, it is because it is normally manufactured with better Peruvian bark than is available in Angola.

It is certain that *água de Inglaterra*, being less cloying due to the wine that disguises the Peruvian bark's bitterness, can be taken in larger doses and more often without provoking nausea. It is for this reason that it may be preferable in those cases in which the debility of the stomach is prone to vomit up its contents, even only light broth. *Água de Inglaterra*, as well as powdered Peruvian bark, often helps loosen the bowels that, because of the weakness of the peristaltic motion of the intestines, may be found to be blocked. Such release is always preferable to that provoked by purgatives.

The vehicle through which the Peruvian bark should be administered is that which, while disguising the Peruvian bark's bitterness, is most agreeable to the palate of the patient. I have observed milk being used as the better vehicle, despite poorly grounded theories and the

---

*Powdered Peruvian bark, two ounces; cold water, twenty-four ounces; allow to infuse for ten to twelve hours and filter. [*Pharmacopoeia . . . Londinensis*, p. 25; *Pharmacopeia Geral*, vol. 2, p. 90.—Ed.]

injurious opposition that has been laid against the use of milk for fevers by the old empirical physicians. This opposition still exists, except in the case of hectic fevers.

In severe attacks of fever, when it is necessary to keep vigil through the night and day in order to take advantage of the remission, Peruvian bark should be administered in milk whey or by infusion, or even in *água de Inglaterra*, as soon as the pulse slows and the body temperature comes down. This is the surest way of moderating or preventing the subsequent paroxysm, because there is no way of being sure whether or not the fever will complete the remission, since it may just slow the symptoms rather than result in complete remission. However, in ordinary fevers and less intense fits there is no need for the same treatment, and we can hope for a whole and long remission.

There are occasions when, as well as loosening the bowels, Peruvian bark will cause such violent diarrhea that their contents, including the Peruvian bark, will be expelled from the anus without any change in its natural state. This symptom can manifest so quickly that it can frighten the physician to see the patient in such distress. However, because this diarrhea is caused by the tonic virtue of the remedy rather than the illness, it is not a bad thing. It can be easily remedied through introducing three or four drops of *thebaic* tincture in each dose of Peruvian bark administered.*

The heat, the affliction, the restlessness, and the many other symptoms that appear during the first paroxysm, get much worse in the second if their remission is neglected; however, if the extension of the remission and the condition of the bowels permit the use of Peruvian bark, this will have a considerable effect on and influence over the subsequent paroxysm.

Remission of the second paroxysm must be exploited in the same way as the first, with another ounce and a half of Peruvian bark. This should also be continued through the third or fourth remissions, until there are no more signs of fever, since with this method the fever never surpasses a fifth paroxysm.

*Tincture of opium. [*Pharmacopoeia ... Londinensis*, p. 100; *Pharmacopeia Geral*, vol. 2, p. 212.—Ed.]

To take advantage of the effects of Peruvian bark, it is necessary for the bowels to be loose, since I have observed that two or three fluxes, or evacuations, every twenty-four hours not only provide the patient with a great deal of relief from the pain of blocked bowels, but also prolong the remission. Laxative enemas, or five or six grains of rhubarb in each dose of Peruvian bark, should be administered until such time as the bowels are able to evacuate.

It is not uncommon for physicians to administer an emetic as soon as the patient has an attack of nausea and vomiting. I have observed this to be perilous, even fatal. The irritation of the bowels increases with such force that they will not respond to any other remedy after the emetic, with the patient dying while in constant spasm and often vomiting bile.

While the bowels are full of yellow bile the patient will certainly vomit repeatedly; however, the ease with which it comes and the quantity of the bile that is expelled distinguishes it from other vomited material. In such cases I normally administer warm water or chamomile tea to cleanse the bowels and relieve the symptom.

If the vomiting does not cease, but rather continues through the remission, I will continue to administer an effervescent saline mix.* This treatment is often vomited up as a result of the patient's repulsion of the salt combined with lemon juice or vinegar; and as the effect of this treatment consists in the tonic virtue of the fixed air released from the salt, it has greater attraction for the vegetable acid with which it is in contact than it has for the fixed air with which it is combined. I will then saturate an amount of pure water with the fixed air, which I then administer to the patient, who will take it without becoming nauseated. The effect of water saturated with fixed air is more effective because the patient can take it in larger doses without vomiting, even with the dose of four ounces being administered each hour.†

---

*Kali, half an eighth; vegetable acid, three spoons: mix, take, and repeat every hour. [*Pharmacopoeia . . . Londinensis*, p. 39; *Pharmacopeia Geral*, vol. 2, p. 181.—Ed.]

†The water which I use is saturated according to the method of Priestley. [Azeredo here recommends the method outlined by Joseph Priestley, in his *Directions for Impregnating Water with Fixed Air: In Order to Communicate to It the Peculiar Spirit and Virtues of Pyrmont Water, and Other Mineral Waters of a Similar Nature* (London: J. Johnson, 1772).—Ed.]

However, often the continuous vomiting will not respond to these treatments. In such cases I will normally add twenty-five drops of thebaic tincture to a saline mix or saturated water, which I will administer occasionally, increasing or reducing the dose according to the urgency of the case and the condition of the patient. The majority of modern writers have recommended the use of a caustic over the epigastric region in similar cases.* I do not doubt the beneficial effect of this remedy, but I have no experience of applying it, as I have always been able to stop the vomiting by using the treatment described above. Five or six drops of *catholic balsam*[70] taken in any manner have often proved successful.

The vomiting can without doubt continue while the bowels are blocked, and because of this I never forget enemas, even when they are not necessary, because they can help reduce the vomiting by increasing the peristaltic movement of the intestines. And how many times has vomiting been caused by the imprudent use of emetics?

We must begin to administer Peruvian bark as soon as the vomiting stops; however, we cannot use it in its pure solid form, because this could produce another bout of vomiting. In this situation I will normally use either a Peruvian bark infusion or *água de Inglaterra*, both of which take effect more quickly.

While the fever is growing I have lately been applying James's powders.[71] Supported by the attestations of Dr. Hunter,† I have administered the powders despite not observing all the benefits described by the author. However, what is certain is that the powders, by provoking sweat and loosening the bowels, provide the patient with some relief; nevertheless, this outcome is not always certain, and often the powders, which are administered in doses of five to eight grains, have absolutely no effect, and when the dose is increased it becomes a strong emetic. Antimony combined with opium will always cause sweating and will

---

*Catharide salve or plaster. [*Pharmacopoeia . . . Londinensis*, p. 139; *Pharmacopeia Geral*, vol. 1, p. 150.—Ed.]

†See Hunter's *Observations on the Diseases of the Army in Jamaica*, p. 114. [Azeredo here refers to John Hunter (d. 1809), *Observations on the Diseases of the Army in Jamaica; and on the Best Means of Preserving the Health of Europeans in That Climate* (London: G. Nicol, 1788), p. 114.—Ed.]

produce the desired relief within a short space of time.* The normal effect of this treatment on these patients is so appreciable that they often ask for it to be repeated as soon as they are affected by another paroxysm.

Headaches are often so painful that the patient becomes desperate. I normally treat such headaches with opium,† and should this fail to bring about the desired relief I will place a caustic on the nape of the neck, a treatment that always works for me.‡ When the headache is not accompanied with a fever, then a cloth soaked in *volatile alkali* [ammonia], and applied to the nape of the neck will provide relief, with the cloth being soaked every time it dries out and reapplied.

With heat and thirst also affecting such patients, I allow them to drink as much cold water as they wish. I believe cold water to be the most appropriate drink for a patient with a fever, and certainly much better than any other drink recommended in the materia medica. While certainly acting as a refrigerant, lemonades are often instantly harmful. They relax the stomach and cause indigestion, bowel pains, intestinal spasms, and even dysenteries. The common view that fever consists of too much heat has served to persuade everyone that any cold remedy is useful in its treatment. I have witnessed many patients being placed in danger while the physician busies himself in applying refrigerants and *antiphlogistics*, or anti-inflammatories, seeking to treat the heat as the cause of the fever. Saltpeter is often useful in the treatment of fevers, not because it is a refrigerant, but because it is a natural salt that can help produce urine and sweat, as is the case with almost all stimulants.

During the fever's abatement, following a violent paroxysm, nothing is more appropriate than a cordial. Wine is the best of these, especially Port, but Madeira is also suitable. I normally administer wine mixed

*Opium tincture, forty drops; antimony wine, thirty drops; simple cinnamon water, one ounce; stir. [See *Pharmacopoeia . . . Londinensis*, p. 100; *Pharmacopeia Geral*, vol. 2, p. 212.—Ed.]

†Opium tincture; thirty drops distilled with a sugar cube. [*Pharmacopoeia . . . Londinensis*, p. 100; *Pharmacopeia Geral*, vol. 2, p. 212.—Ed.]

‡Cantharide salve, half ounce. [*Pharmacopoeia . . . Londinensis*, p. 139; *Pharmacopeia Geral*, vol. 1, p. 150.—Ed.]

with an equal amount of water and make the patient take it frequently in small doses so as not to provoke vomiting.

Since the stomach will not be able to accept either food or wine while the fever is rising, in order to help patients keep their strength, it is important that this be administered as soon as the remission begins and during the intervals between doses of Peruvian bark. Soups made from chicken, barley, rice, and bread crumbs mixed with wine should be fed to the patient in the intervals between doses of Peruvian bark.

It is often better not to give Peruvian bark on an empty stomach. Since the patient generally knows what is best in this respect, unless his choice is clearly harmful to him, the patient should be allowed to make this decision. This will help the Peruvian bark reach and remain in the stomach, which will help the patient accept repeated doses of the treatment.

When after two or more paroxysms the patient is exhausted, he should be given more wine and food than Peruvian bark. I have observed that it makes little or no difference in these circumstances. It is essential, therefore, to provide the patient from time to time with a small amount either of the food he desires or that which is chosen by the physician. If there should be a break in this regular administration, no matter how brief, the patient will gradually fade and the pulse will diminish until it completely disappears, as if all strength has been completely exhausted by the preceding paroxysm.

It is difficult to determine the positive quantity of wine and food the patient must consume in these circumstances. I have been guided by the following observations: if the wine and food is not to the patient's liking and is rejected, then it is rarely beneficial; should it increase the patient's heat and anxiety it will never produce a good result; however, if the patient likes it, he can be given a pint of diluted wine for every twenty-four hours.

Here I will not speak of the nervous fevers that tend to be caused by the weak reaction of a heart that cannot overcome spasm,* the only

---

*Typhus sive febris nervosa, febris contagiosa, calor parum auctus, pulsus parvus, debilis, frequens, urina parum mutata, sensorii functiones, plurimum turbata, vires multum imminutae. [Typhoid fever or nervous and contagious fever; low temperature; weak,

cure for which is large amounts of wine. However, great care must be taken to avoid drunkenness, which is only capable of causing new and more dangerous paroxysms.

Should the patient continue to experience thirst, there is nothing more satisfying than cold water; however, I tend to place a piece of toasted bread in the water. The majority of physicians I have met like to administer sour or acidic liquors to quench the thirst; however, they are wrong. While sour and acidic beverages will quench the patient's thirst, after a while they will produce anxiety and stomach pains. Dryness in the mouth can be relieved with the occasional spoonful of tinned tamarind.

When the paroxysm is accompanied with deliria, coma, or lethargy, I believe nothing works with greater promptitude and efficacy than a caustic[72] to the nape of the neck. I am convinced that the beneficial effect of this treatment lies in the stimulation caused by the cantharides absorbed into the lymphatic vessels, rather than in the excretion produced by the wound. Consequently, as soon as it seems the patient is not receiving any benefit from the application of the caustic, I place powdered cantharides on the wound to ensure greater stimulation. In order to heal the wound I completely ignore basil, which only serves to increase the pain the patient is suffering. Once the discharge of fluid and the removal of the caustic occur, I cover the wound without separating the cuticle with a white wax, or with unsalted butter; since the discharge is useless, there is no use for irritating patches.

However, when the delirium is not dangerous and the lethargy not profound, I find there to be advantages in administering small doses of opium every two hours. These same doses have often resulted in complete remission from fever.

Flatulence, which comes from the stomach and the intestines, often causes a tumescence in the bowels to swell so much that it causes pain throughout the body. This flatulence can be expelled with laxative enemas or, should that fail, with two or three drops of peppermint

---

feeble and rapid pulse; nearly unaltered urine, highly disturbed sensory functions, extremely diminished strength. — Trans.] [See Cullen (1780), vol. 2, p. 71; and (1784), vol. 1, p. 112, note 5. — Ed.]

oil taken with a lump of sugar, or two or even three spoons of camphor julep, which will normally expel the trapped air. The administration of Peruvian bark must always continue while these remedies are attempted.

I believe bloodletting during these fevers to be entirely pernicious. Use of the lancet has had some disastrous consequences when applied by those who have only read Sydenham. I have learned that while the loss of even a small amount of blood may not do apparent harm, it is also of no benefit whatsoever. I venture to state that more fevers are cured when they are completely ignored than are cured by bloodletting. It is the treatment administered by physicians that normally make illnesses dangerous in Africa: physicians who cling to a particular system and who are unable to choose or think in a way that is different from their routine. In the rare cases in which it has proved successful, it is not because of its precision or utility.

Headaches are almost always relieved by scarifying the nape of the neck, which I do because it is faster acting than the application of a caustic. However, should these pains be accompanied by delirium, unconsciousness, or any other symptom that suggests a reduction in brain activity, then I prefer to apply a caustic. It is better than scarification because, while the effect of the former [scarification] may be vigorous, together they are slow, and it [the caustic] will be more effective and decisive. In these cases I will apply both treatments so that I am not reliant on just one that may fail. The use of scarification has become excessive in the country, so much so that patients have been known to administer the treatment to themselves, without the opinion of any physician. In this way everywhere and every day inappropriate scarifications are being made, which can aggravate illnesses that are by nature benign.

Obstructions must be assessed both during the rise of the fever and after. The idea that Peruvian bark is the cause of this in patients with fevers is completely wrong. In the past, physicians tended to confuse the effect with the cause. How many complaints are there in which copious use is made of Peruvian bark and no obstructions ever appear? And how many times have there been fevers when no Peruvian bark has been administered? I am convinced Peruvian bark is incapable of causing obstructions, and I will continue to use it to treat fevers regardless of how large any obstructions may be. During paroxysms, each day I will embrocate the obstructed part of the entrail with an eighth part of mercurial unguent, as this seems to me to be the best ameliorative that can be applied externally. However, once the fever has stopped rising, I will then use a range of internally applied treatments for obstructions, the best of which I have discovered to be mercury, ammoniac gum, and hemlock.* Because I have had success with it, the administration of large doses of opium is the only treatment in which I have any faith in those cases where either tetanus or lockjaw survives a fever.† I combine the opium with Peruvian bark when the fever goes into remission. The doses of opium must be administered every hour until the spasms stop. I know the doses of opium that are normally administered are not enough to produce the desired effect. In cases of tetanus, opium can be administered in very large doses without any danger whatsoever. I myself have administered an ounce of thebaic tincture every half hour during a fever that was accompanied with a violent tetanus, just to ensure that the patient had an hour of rest, and I repeated the same doses to secure a similar period of rest, as we will see below.

Nosebleeds, being normally favorable and not worthy of attention, can sometimes become so excessive that they place the patient's life in peril. However, they are easily treated with trivial medicines, such as by applying cold water to the head or the feet; by placing the hands in warm water; by administering a hip bath of cold water; by the application of a dry cloth, or one soaked in vinegar or wine spirit, to the nostrils, or a swab soaked in egg white, or [in] equal parts sugar and powdered alum or potash applied to the nostrils. However, should these fail (as has happened), a light purgative of Glauber's salt with manna and a caustic to the nape of the neck will always stop the bleeding.

---

*Ammoniac gum, one eighth. Soap, four *scruples* [an archaic unit of measure used by apothecaries; approximately 1.2 grams—Ed.]. Stir and form into pills. Dose of five pills. In addition, extract of hemlock, one ounce. Powdered hemlock leaves, as much as is necessary, form into pills, dose five grains.

†Tincture of opium, one eighth in a glass of wine each hour. [*Pharmacopoeia . . . Londinensis*, p. 100; *Pharmacopeia Geral*, vol. 2, p. 212.—Ed.]

The pains in the legs and the thighs will be alleviated and diminish with the application of some ointment.* I have sometimes found it useful to wrap the legs and thighs in baize cloths soaked in hot water. I prefer this method to bathing, which I believe can be harmful to patients as it saps their strength. Opium does not provide any relief for these pains; however, opium can be useful if the pains occur as the fever is rising, as it can relieve the fever and lead to remission.

In cases of hydrocephalus, caustics can be applied to the neck, the forehead, and the temples. Calomel can also be administered to stimulate the absorbent vessels; however, I have nothing to say about this because the fever will decide before the mercury is able to take effect.

To fortify their patients, physicians will normally use those remedies called alexipharmics, or antidotes, and cordials; however, I have nothing to say about them because I never need to make use of them when I have good Peruvian bark and fine wine.

Contrary to common belief, while caustics can increase brain activity, in no way can they reduce the fever. I have applied caustics in several violent paroxysms and have never been able to ascertain whether they have ever brought down a fever.

Since the waste product of the caustic is completely useless, it must be used for as short a time as possible, because its continued use will weaken the patient and the muscles in the area to which it is applied. I have seen some sores caused by the application of caustic patches turn into ulcers and then turn gangrenous, which is fatal.

Red Peruvian bark is not as effective as white Peruvian bark, because it generally causes bowel pains and vomiting. Common people, supported by many physicians, who are unaccustomed to seeking the truth, fear Peruvian bark as a hot and caustic treatment according to the old way of thinking. Because of this they avoid using it, seeking instead to treat fevers with lemonades and sodas. Those who do administer it seek to refrigerate after using it, and attribute to it all the eruptions and scabs that normally appear in the wake of cured fevers. This prejudice can

---

*Ammonium liniment, or soap liniment. [*Pharmacopoeia . . . Londinensis*, p. 151; *Pharmacopeia Geral*, vol. 2, p. 172.—Ed.]

still be found among some physicians who wish to be called modern, and unprejudiced.

In continuous fevers, which are only recognizable by the weakness of the pulse, higher temperatures, and sometimes light headaches, because the patient stays on his feet and continues with his daily tasks, I have found no treatment more effective than hot baths. Hot baths help the patient drift into sleep with a moderate sweat, which proves the spasm of the skin has relaxed. In this I follow the method used by Ebenezer Gilchrist,* and I find the fevers that resist all anti-spasm treatments will respond to baths in which the whole body is immersed, and four or five repetitions is enough to complete the treatment. Patients should remain in the bath for no more than fifteen minutes, for to do so would increase their debility, which would prevent the effective treatment of the fever, and would thereby turn harmful.

*See Gilchrist, appendix upon the usage of bath on fevers. [Ebenezer Gilchrist, appendix "Concerning Bathing in Fevers," in *The Use of Sea Voyages in Medicine* (London: A. Millar, D. Wilson, and T. Durham, 1756).—Ed.] [Ebenezer Gilchrist (1707–74), Scottish physician.—Trans.]

Essay on Intermittent Fevers

I have no need to provide a new historical narrative of intermittent fevers because their symptoms are the same as those already outlined above for remittent fevers. The proximate and remote causes are also the same, so for this reason a new exposition is pointless work that will only increase the size of the book with repetitions. Consequently I will pass directly to treatments, where perhaps there will appear some developments that will be of interest.

Cure

Quotidian intermittent fevers[73] should be treated immediately with an emetic. It will often cure everything if taken half an hour before any fever begins to take hold, preventing the fever from rising anew. It is quite natural for the shock of the emetic to occur at precisely the moment when the spasm returns, and a new fit begins; it stimulates the fibers and restricts the spasm from forming. In addition, it evacuates the intestines, making them ready to receive tonics during the subsequent intermissions, in those cases in which it does not halt the fever.

With the second attack or paroxysm of fever having begun after the patient's bowels have been evacuated, it is recommended that we wait for its intermission, when an ounce of Peruvian bark can be administered. Should the fever not respond to the emetic it will quickly respond to the Peruvian bark and the patient will stabilize. Quite often, however, fevers will not be cured with only one ounce of Peruvian bark, and a new resurgence will take place. In this case, the patient should be given another ounce of Peruvian bark during the next intermission, and this should be continued until the fits begin to lose force.

For the fevers to pause there is no need to seek assistance from medicine because the increased action of the heart will put an end to the spasm and cause the body to sweat. The cold water the patient drinks will not only cool him down, but will also contribute to the diaphoresis that helps with the fever's abatement. However, should the attack be much more violent than previously, I will administer opium in order to prevent the fever becoming remittent,* which is not unknown. In this case, as soon as the patient begins to sweat I will administer a double dose of Peruvian bark, even two ounces, but only if there is an intermission, and only if the stomach will tolerate it. Few quotidian intermittent fevers will resist this treatment.

I have noted that when Peruvian bark is taken by patients whose bowels and stomach have not been evacuated it afflicts them by hardening the guts without preventing the fit. In order to prevent this from happening when the first emetic has not functioned well as a cathartic, I will administer a purgative immediately after the emetic, and before administering any Peruvian bark.† After this, the tonic will have a natural effect by being better able to reach the walls of the intestines.

Despite the marvelous virtue of Peruvian bark, there are still quotidian intermittent fevers that resist it. I have been obliged to resort to other treatments in order to provide my patients with relief. The lack of Peruvian bark, which is a common problem in Luanda, was the reason I was forced to find some other means of suppressing the fever. I did not fail to avail myself of these examinations and tests.

I found *nux vomica* to have equal, or even superior, benefit to that of Peruvian bark for the treatment of quotidian intermittent fevers. I later demonstrated its beneficial effects both within the hospital and outside, and all the physicians began, by necessity, prescribing it, and now it is prescribed for examinations. The same people making use of the prescriptions in their possession now take them without fear and without the advice of the physician. This treatment, which was not known in Luanda before my arrival, is now commonplace. During an intermission it can be administered in doses of one-eighth of an ounce.‡

---

*Thirty drops of opium tincture. Half pound of almond milk. One-eighth ounce of antimony syrup; stir.

†One ounce of manna. Two ounces of tamarind. Half ounce of cream of tartar. Eight ounces of hot water. Stir.

‡One-eighth of *nux vomica*. As much common syrup as necessary. Form into pills. [The active ingredient in nux vomica is trace amounts of strychnine.—Ed.]

At times I have combined it with some bitters, and now it seems to work with greater efficacy.*

Like all treatments, this can often fail, which drove me to seek another that would work in such cases. I used one that, while more violent and a lethal venom, is at the same time one of the most effective and useful antidotes to quotidian intermittent fevers. The name of this remedy is white arsenic. When administered during a perfect intermission, it never fails to cure all fevers. It never produces its perilous side effects when applied prudently. I have given it to many people of both sexes and of all ages, and I have not yet had even one failure. A dose of two grains in each intermission is enough for a robust man,† and the fevers are unfailingly defeated with the second or sometimes third repetition of this remedy, which is as safe as it is sound.

Some time ago I was persuaded that *tertian* and *quartian* fevers[74] cannot be cured with Peruvian bark, or, rather, they can resist its effects for months or even years.

Experience has also shown me that they can resist *nux vomica* and white arsenic. These failings obliged me to put an infinite number of treatments into practice, and after some years of frustrated experimentation I discovered one that is as effective with these fevers as white arsenic is with quotidian fevers. The outer shell of the coconut, that which is used for brushes, which is cooked and drunk on days free of fever, never fails to cure these fevers.‡ These results had already been found by others, to whom I communicated their effectiveness, and who found in them the same beneficial effects. I can confirm that while I have *nux vomica*, white arsenic, coconut shell, and laxatives and emetics, then I have no fear of intermittent fevers, and I often even dispense with Peruvian bark altogether.

---

*One-eighth of *nux vomica*. Half eighth of powdered gentian root. As much common syrup as necessary. Form into pills.

†Two grains of white arsenic; six grains of tartarized kali—grind together and mix. Add a touch of rose extract; form into pills (two).

‡Ten ounces of the crushed coconut shell. Four quarts of pure water boiled until reduced to two quarts. Leave for three hours, then strain.

Essay on the Dysenteries of Angola

Dysentery is, in my view, "pyrexia with tenesmus, gripes, anorexia, nausea, frequent mucous or bloody evacuations with few feces or, more often than not, without them."[75]

Physicians ordinarily confuse dysentery with diarrhea, which is very different both in their proximate and remote causes and cure. They must be distinguished in order to treat them without killing the patient, as I see all too often through the application of remedies for dysentery that are inappropriate and even pernicious.

The dysentery that I am about to describe is the same as that described by Sydenham, Pringle, Baker,[76] Hunter, and others. However, I have observed some symptoms of which they make no mention, perhaps because these are peculiar to African dysenteries, or because they did not witness the same complications. Since I am outlining a method of treatment that is more perfect than those that have heretofore emerged, I will refer only to my observations and avoid citing authorities, in order to stay brief and not repeat that which others have said. I will describe facts as they have been witnessed in my practice.

History of Dysentery

There is a powerful connection between remittent fevers and dysentery, so much so that one can easily become the other and they often complicate each other. Dysentery often ends in fever, and more often than not, fevers will end in dysentery.

During some seasons dysentery is so commonplace that it seems epidemic; however, during the hot months, which in Angola are from October to May, dysentery is more commonplace and more deadly. I have not yet been able to discover the extent to which heat contributes to this complaint.

Dysentery often appears as the result of a revolution of the gut that leads to some gentle pains in the umbilical region that end with some evacuation of the bowels. However, while the patient wants to evacuate, for a long time he will be tormented by tenesmus and will eventually produce a little mucus[77] resembling egg whites in which there are spots of blood. The anus becomes inflamed, and the patient feels excessively hot in the belly, with a heat in the gut like that of a pepper.

These symptoms increase until pyrexia takes over, the mouth becomes bitter and the tongue turns white, anorexia appears, the body weakens and the spirit fades.

At the beginning there is normally a copious watery discharge and some excrement, but the following day, or even before, only a small amount of watery fecal matter is passed, while the patient suffers ongoing tenesmus and griping in the guts. Dysenteric fluxes, or discharges, differ from natural evacuations in their intolerable cadaverous stench, which is very different from normal, and which is perhaps the result of a decay that has already begun in the intestines.

Flatulence is one of the most common symptoms of dysentery and almost always indicates the existence of the complaint. The belly swells and the accumulation of gas in the intestines increases the pain and causes continual turmoil.

As soon as dysentery progresses, the patient will also experience urine retention and pains in the bladder and urethra. The prognosis at this point is fatal. The retentions often torment patients so much they forget their dysentery and seek only to alleviate the symptom, believing that by doing so they will be able to restore their health.

However, the extent to which the dysentery increases, the tenesmus diminishes; the flatulence decreases, the belly shrinks, the muscles of the abdomen almost meet the spine, the anus opens and the sphincter loses its ability to contract, and the flow of urine is no more than a needle of water that the patient does not sense leaving his body.

The patient being reduced to this lamentable condition, with a mouth that is completely dry and which cannot be moistened, with an extraordinary and constant thirst, with a corpse-like countenance with deeply gaunt eyes, drawn cheeks, and sharpened nose, the body gives off an insufferable and corrupt odor, the pulse is fast and weak, and the extremities completely cold and humid. All these symptoms indicate the illness is incurable and death is near.

I have discovered some more particular symptoms that normally appear a few hours before the patient dies. On many occasions the dysentery has progressed, the patient does not evacuate at all, but confesses to feeling better and free of illness. This reduction in or suppression of evacuations is always a sign of approaching death, that is, it is proof there is no peristaltic activity in the intestines and that the patient has lost sensitivity and vital power.

On other occasions the dysentery continues to gradually wear down the patient's strength until he is without pulse and cold in the extremities, all the time saying he is feeling better and speaking without noticing any difficulty or fearing anything. The absence of a pulse in this situation is a certain indication that the patient does not have long to live.

The end of dilated and chronic dysenteries can be seen in the patient's eyes. Because the eyes have lost their natural movement, the patient will begin to squint, flicking from one unmoving eye to the other with dilated pupils. The patient will remain in this condition for some time, until he dies.

In some cases of dysentery I have watched patients die following a small and transient delirium that made me wonder if this experience had not shown me a disheartening and unexpected consequence that I would always carry with me.

Often there is a vomiting in which a great deal of black and green bile is brought up. Such patients may spend two or three days in this condition, or sometimes much less; however, they do not normally escape from it.

The most common symptom, which always indicates gangrene in the intestines, is the hiccups. These will affect the patient for three or more days prior to death, and nothing can relieve them. Often they will stop, allowing the patient some rest, but they will return, which some physicians have thought is the effect of some remedy they had applied, but in fact it is merely the effect of nature and the same illness. At times the hiccups persecute the patient right up to the moment he dies, while at other times they will stop some hours before death.

The blood found in the fluxes does not normally appear until the end and therefore is neither a dire symptom nor indicative of the gravity of the complaint. It is clear that sometimes there is a profusion of blood. In patients suffering from hemorrhoids who are struck by dysentery, there is often so much blood it frightens both the patient and the physician. Dysentery can cause hemorrhage when there is already a disposition for it in the system.

Since hemorrhoids are often accompanied with tenesmus, it can often be difficult to determine the nature of the complaint; however, if we carefully examine all the symptoms, we will seldom or never be wrong. Tenesmus in dysentery is accompanied by bowel pains, while with hemorrhoids the pain is in the anus. The blood from bleeding caused by dysentery will be mixed with the contents of the intestines, while the blood from hemorrhoidal bleeding is pure. Hemorrhoids cause vertigo, pains in the loins, and *tubercles*[78] in the anus, while dysentery causes abdominal gripes, anorexia, and frequent bowel fluxes or evacuations.

One symptom that almost always occurs with this complaint, and of which few have spoken, is that as soon as the patient swallows something, whether solid or liquid, he will immediately need to evacuate, so that he feels that whatever is ingested passes directly through the bowels to reach the anus. This sensation is so powerful that the patient will not be convinced otherwise and will refrain from eating or drinking, fearing only that the food will pass through the body immediately. This symptom is proof of the irritability of the intestines, when the movements in the bowels caused by the ingestion of food spread immediately through the intestines to the anus.

Some dysenteries last only a few days, while others last much longer. Those that are serious do not kill the patient immediately, nor do they leave the patient free of all symptoms, because such patients often experience simple diarrhea that is vexatious and which can endure for months or years without responding to treatment, until either nature wins out or it turns into dysentery, which is difficult to avoid.

If the patient is fortunate to overcome the complaint, he will remain in a most deplorably weakened and cachexic[79] condition. The legs will for some time be edematous, the body destitute of flesh, the stomach will suffer continuous dyspepsias, despondency, and looseness, and weariness will affect every movement and activity. This same debility can be observed in those dysenteries that last for only eight days, which shows just how much they attack the system in general.

Anal prolapse has been a consequence of dysentery when the tenesmus is continuous and strong. This keeps the patient restless and in pain all day and awake all night. The body's waste contains a great deal of blood because of the swelling of the closed part of the anus, which prevents the contents of the intestines from leaving the body. In this case the relaxation of the sphincter is hasty, and gangrene in the rectal intestine appears quickly.

I have observed that after gangrene sets in and the way is opened, hardened balls of fecal matter exit floating on the fluid that makes up the waste. These scybala[80] are not completely round; rather, they are irregular, as if they had been deposited between the alveoli and circular folds within the bowels and retained because there was no way of expelling them; that is to say, because of spasms in these folds.

At other times I have seen material of different color, consistency, and quality in the waste. Sometimes there is mucus, while at others there is pus, and others still a putrid *sanies*.[81]

I have also often found *sebaceous*[82] matter resembling the pieces of cheese described by Pringle and others, and which they call *corpora pinguia*, or body fat.[83] I believe this material to be mucus that often appears in waste, hardened by the heat in the body, long retention, and lack of movement.

I cannot decide whether dysentery is or is not contagious. However, if I must judge according to its remote and proximate causes, if I must convince myself of what experience has taught me, I am inclined to state that it is not contagious, despite the opinions of many authors who have written about this complaint. I think it is very difficult to reach their same conclusion when the evidence of contagion is not clear, let alone decisive. With epidemic diseases, it is easy to confuse an effect with a general widespread cause that the disease spreads. It is true that we have observed that some of the effluvia produced by rotting animals can quickly attack the intestines and cause diarrhea. However, I have not yet seen these substances cause real dysentery. Moreover, while these substances increase the peristaltic movement of the intestines (which is the proximate cause of diarrhea), they cannot produce dysentery, the proximate cause of which, as we shall see below, consists of the constriction of the colon and rectum.

Proximate Cause

I will now inquire into a more obscure point. Knowledge of the proximate cause of dysentery has until now been very limited, and involved conjecture and hypotheses. In past times the common view was that the proximate cause of dysentery was a material acridity that, when introduced to or generated within the intestines, caused pains, tenesmus, and bowel evacuations. However, this opinion lost support when Pringle, seeking to prove that the human body is continually decomposing, suggested that the immediate cause of dysentery was a putrid fermentation within the general blood mass. However, Pringle's ideas had no longevity. There is no better way to discover the truth than through experience. Ever since Hewson has analyzed the blood, we have been certain that it does not contain this noxious matter, nor are there any signs of decomposition; thus, the view once held as the truth has been cast aside.

Recalling what Thomas Bartholin[84] had observed in the excrement of patients with dysentery, Carl Linnaeus[85] sought to prove that the cause of dysentery is live dust mites that exist within the colonic and rectal intestines, where they cause damage. Physicians find Linnaeus's opinion hard to believe, and no one defends it from the serious objections raised against it. Observations tell us there are dysenteries caused by the application of cold to the body, while there is not the least suspicion of mites being introduced into or produced by the intestines.

There is nothing that can cast a clearer light and provide a more perfect idea of the proximate cause of dysentery than the dissection of corpses. This is how from the earliest days of medicine we have discovered most of the causes of illnesses of which we now have knowledge; it is how we escape from the labyrinth of hypotheses and conjectures and make clear our mistakes and misunderstandings. The following is what I have learned through dissections.

On opening the abdominal cavity[86] and separating the *omentum*,[87] one is immediately presented with an irregularly contracted colon that is a deeper red than other intestines. The rest of the internal organs within the cavity remain in their natural state. Sometimes I have found the inferior part of the omentum to be dark blue, which I am persuaded is accidental and has no connection whatsoever with the illness. On dissecting a portion of the small intestines, they appear to be in perfect condition, with their *tunics*, or outer membranes, appearing uninjured and their *mesentery*[88] showing no sign of damage. However, on dissecting a section of the colon and performing a detailed examination of its tunics, I find the nature of the complaint becomes clear. In it we find tubercles in the form of pustules that appear in varying amounts and in different states. Some of these tubercles are large, hard, and red, while others are small and dark; however, inside they are completely white and made of a substance that appears similar to fragments of cheese. They are situated between the villous[89] and muscular intestinal *tunics*, or membranes. The contraction observed in the colon is much more irregular in the rectum, the tunics of which are much larger and softer than the others. The villous tunic was destroyed and converted into that mucus which accompanies the fluxes. In the muscular tunic I noted some small ulcers between the tubercles, which were discovered only after taking care to clean out the mucus and bile, of which there is a great deal. When squeezed, the tubercles expelled a fluid that appeared to be pus mixed with blood. The bladder was completely contracted and the ileum[90] greatly inflamed. This is what I have observed in every dissection of victims of dysentery.

Pringle mentioned gangrene in the villous intestinal tunic, but I have never encountered it. I have often found some parts of the colon and rectum to be black, but rather than attributing this to gangrene I put it down to extravasated blood. I do not doubt there is gangrene in the muscular and nerve tunics, or membranes, that pass to the villi, but this is no more than a mere hypothesis.

Should dissections show me a spasm and constriction of the colon and rectum, should we concede there is a link between dysentery and fever, the proximate cause of which consists of a spasm induced by indirect debility, then I would be correctly persuaded that the proximate cause of dysentery is the colonic and rectal spasms induced by their own weakness.

However, how can this spasm affect only these two intestines? The remote cause that it produced affects only the colon and the rectum.

This step is very difficult to follow. However, were I to look to the laws of nature, were I to search for an analogy, were I to have to believe the facts and the experiences, then I know the objections have no weight, despite being unable to explain *a priori* the acts of nature. Each day, experience shows me that generic causes produce partial complaints; therefore, why can a generic cause not be capable of producing a partial spasm? I see that a cause applied to the body in general produces abscesses on or inflammation of the tonsils, pleurisy, hepatitis, etc., so why can it not produce spasms in the colon and the rectum with the cause applied to everything?

We know that in order to function, first the precipitating causes need to have the proper predisposing conditions. If the predisposing conditions are only partially available, then the effect will only be partial because only a part will receive the precipitating cause. No matter the generic cause applied to the system, it will affect only the colonic and rectal intestines if they are disposed to be affected.

Retained scybala, bowel pains, tenesmus, and urine retention are clear proof of spasm. Morgagni[91] noted that bleeding is more a consequence of the dilation of the vessels that proceeded from the spasms in the neighboring fibers than a result of the rupture of these same vessels. However, as a result of the dissections, I am always convinced the blood seeps from the small ulcers found in the intestines. Yet, is this constriction, caused by the general cause, that which produces the ulcers? If so, then Morgagni's opinion, while wrong, is at least more agreeable.

The spasm, which continues for want of a suitable remedy, or because of the upheaval of the illness, will eventually succumb to asthenic relaxation, which is the onset of gangrene. As a result, the tenesmus will cease; the pains and flatulence will diminish as soon as the relaxation begins or the spasm declines. Nevertheless, the excretions will continue as a consequence of the intestines and sphincter losing their tone and vital power.

Remote Causes

Remote causes are those that, when applied to the body, induce abatements and spasms in the colon and rectum. Their fibers are more susceptible and amenable to receive these agitations. I am almost certain that the motivating causes leading to dysentery are the same as those leading to fever. As with fevers, it is certain that the body's atmospheric heat will increase sharply.

The excessive consumption of strong adulterated spirits, the exposure of the feet to humidity, a lack of cleanliness, indigestible food, and whimsical passions of the soul have all evidently produced dysentery. Similarly, this effect can also come from using powerful purgatives.

It is not yet possible to determine whether the effluvia from stagnant and polluted waters can also lead to dysentery, as it is known they cause fevers. However, since dysentery almost always appears before, during, or after fever, and since their proximate and remote causes are the same, I am inclined to the view that these effluents also cause dysentery when the intestines are predisposed to it, just as they produce fevers when the skin is so predisposed.

Cure

Dysentery must be treated immediately, because the remedies available to overcome or mitigate the complaint will become useless and ineffective with the passing of time. As soon as it appears I administer a light emetic that will almost always result in an evacuation, both because the intestines are so disposed and because I combine it with some absorbent earth.* The patients generally receive some relief with this, particularly when there is too much bile in the stomach, or when they are nauseated. Ipecacuanha,[92] as is usually supposed, has no particular virtue, [and] has the same effect as antimony. I often mix the two and

---

*Tartarized antimony, one grain; manna, one ounce; white magnesium, half an eighth; hot water, three ounces; stir. [*Pharmacopoeia . . . Londinensis*, p. 53; *Pharmacopeia Geral*, vol. 2, p. 131. — Ed.]

administer this in such a dose that will function as a cathartic.* I have administered doses of antimony that are high enough to cause nausea, but have never encountered any benefits.

The following day I repeat the same emetic because I have found a single dose is rarely enough to complete the treatment. Moreover, it is important to repeat the dose in order not to lose time, despite the fact the patient might seem fine. On the night after the second emetic has been administered, I will give a dose of opium.† This will normally cure all dysenteries caught as soon as they appear.

Quite often the complaint will not submit to this initial treatment, so it is important to continue administering remedies. Now that the patient's strength has been sapped, the administration of emetics becomes dangerous. At this point I administer an antiphlogistic purgative. One ounce of any of the neutral salts combined with an ounce of manna dissolved in a quart of hot water is a sufficient purgative.‡ The laxative can be helped by making the patient take chicken or beef soup, tea, or any other diluent of the patient's choice.

As soon as the patient begins to evacuate, the bowel pains and tenesmus will reduce. Following this beneficial evacuation, a single dose of opium during the night will almost always result in a cure.§ The purgative will stop the spasm and provide relief, while the opium will prolong both benefits.

Several purgatives have been recommended by different authors. Glauber's salt, cathartic salt, soluble tartar, senna infusions, castor oil, or any other similar purgative can be used according to the constitution of the patient. Cullen refused to use rhubarb because it is an astringent dangerous in the case of dysentery. I have used it only occasionally and am unable to decide whether its astringency obstructs the treatment. As in all things, I prefer to administer it, combining it with mercury

---

*Ipecacuanha, half an eighth. Tartarized antimony, one grain. Hot water, three ounces: stir.

†Refined pure opium, one grain. Rose conserve, as much as necessary; form into pills.

‡Vitriolic soda or vitriolic magnesium. [*Pharmacopoeia . . . Londinensis*, p. 44.—Ed.]

§Tincture of opium, twenty-five drops. Water of nutmeg, one ounce; stir.

according to Pringle's method.* From this mixture emerges a mild purgative that is just right for dysentery. Perhaps the mercury alters the rhubarb and increases its purgative qualities.

All irritant purgatives are harmful, even fatal, because they increase bowel pains and tenesmus. I have seen some very deadly consequences from the use of jalapa and scammony in a similar complaint.

Only in less serious cases, a single purgative is capable of slowing the progress of the illness, because in serious cases the pains and tenesmus will return as soon as the purgative has ceased its effect. In such cases I will repeat the same purgative the next day and will repeat this on the third day without giving it any respite. I know the patient will not be weakened by the operation of repeatedly administered purgatives, since these seek to provide relief from pain and tenesmus. It should be noted that the patient soon distinguishes between the movements caused by the purgative and those caused by the complaint. Some physicians are convinced of the need for purgatives in this complaint, and used to administer them on alternate days in order to provide the patient with a period of rest. However, this is a mistake, because on the day of rest the patient will continue to evacuate in consequence of the illness. In addition, the fluxes proceeding from the illness are more violent and weaken the patient more than the purgatives. Finally, the illness will progress when time is thus wasted.

Where I have found purgatives to produce no relief I will not abandon them, nor will I begin administering opium, because I am sure that it would be extremely dangerous to give this before the constriction of the intestines has been eliminated by the purgatives.

There is no matter in the practice of medicine on which authors are more divided than in the use of opium in the treatment of dysentery. In many cases, Sydenham has entrusted the entire cure to it, while others of equal authority totally condemn its use. Pringle recommends caution, and counsels its administration only after a favorable evacuation, which means it should only be given at the end of the second day following

*Rhubarb, half an eighth. Calomel, ten grains. Mucilage of Arabic gum, as much as is necessary. Form into pills. [See Pringle, *Observations on Diseases of the Army*, note 89, p. 262.—Ed.]

the first evacuation. I am greatly convinced by Cullen when he says the failure to administer a purgative at the onset of the illness is what makes the later administration of opium necessary. Constant practice has taught me that the immediate beneficial effects of opium are misleading and of short duration when it is administered inopportunely.

Opium administered at any time, and while the patient is in any condition, will immediately ease any pain, reduce fluxes, and let the patient sleep. However, once it wears off the pains will return, the fluxes will increase, and the patient's strength will dissipate. I believe that when opium is given before the intestinal spasms are stopped by the purgatives, it will increase the same spasms as a consequence of the indirect debility remaining after its initial effect wears off. Opium will diminish the growing activity of the intestines excited by constrictions, and will make the nerves insensitive to the pain caused by the spasm; however, it will not remove the spasm, since this is induced by a debility for which the opium is responsible.

However, as soon as the patient feels some relief, as a consequence of the first, second, or third purgative, then a dose of opium in the evening is very useful, not only because it prolongs the beneficial effects of the laxative, but because it also rests the patient, giving him the strength to bear the effects of the next day's purgative, should it prove necessary.

Some physicians will mix opium with emetics or purgatives. This has produced good results in some cases of chronic dysentery. However, I always prefer to alternate between them and administer them separately, since opium always hinders the effect of the purgative and emetic. I am entirely indifferent as to whether opium should be administered as a liquid or a solid, although this has been the subject of some rather irrelevant debate.

The purgatives must be repeated when the illness is very violent. However, at times the complaint is such that it will not respond, which will lead to a weakening of the patient's strength to such an extent that there can be no advantage gained by their continued administration. In such cases I will frequently use ipecacuanha mixed with Peruvian bark, or even rhubarb mixed with Peruvian bark.*

*Peruvian bark infusion, three ounces. Marcela tea, one ounce. Ipecacaunha, rhubarb, one scruple. Poppy syrup, one ounce: stir and take three spoonfuls every two hours.

Bowel pains, which are almost always violent, can be relieved with the use of hip baths, which when repeated are almost always effective in reducing spasm. However, when the pains are very great, these baths provide only momentary relief. I have discovered that cantharides tincture[93] in an ointment applied to the abdomen is not only highly effective in removing the pain, but it even reduces the inflammation of the intestines.* This quick remedy I discovered has greatly advanced the treatment of dysentery because it can be repeated with the frequency the illness demands without causing any discomfort, which is certainly not true of other treatments.

On many occasions I have applied the same caustics to the abdomen; however, I have never found this to have the same immediate effect as the cantharis ointment. Perhaps because, unlike the caustic vesicatoria,[94] the ointment does not cause blistering and can consequently be repeated several times; thus, it allows a greater amount of the cantharis to be absorbed. Additionally, the caustic vesicatoria affects the urinary tract, which can cause damage with this illness, both because there is already a disposition for a similar attack, since we have seen that one of its more powerful symptoms is urine retention; and because the part on which it must be applied is close to the bladder, the effect therefore will be greater. I have found the ointment to produce none of these effects.

On the days of rest, during which the patient is not purged, enemas are very useful and often are enough to complete the cure. Whenever the purgatives cannot be used by the patient, owing to his own weakness, I will administer the enemas. The antiphlogistics and anodynes are the most appropriate.† I give preference to those made from milk, both for their simplicity and for the pain-relieving properties that are natural to them.

Following the first attack of dysentery, the illness will become chronic. This consists of repeated pains and periodic evacuations. In this condition the patient will have two or three good days before the illness returns.

---

*Cantharides tincture, two scruples. Laurel oil, one ounce. Form into a liniment and repeat every three hours.

†Barley water, ten ounces. Poppy heads, one ounce; boil until it reduces to six ounces, strain, and then add two egg whites.

With the patient's strength being worn down every day, the muscles begin to waste, the body gets thinner, and the fever rises. The complaint now consists of looseness in the bowels. This can then be called another illness, for which other treatments are appropriate. Its proximate cause is the overwhelming debility induced by the indirect stimulus: dysentery. It is a second complaint caused by the first, in the same way chronic rheumatism is caused by acute rheumatism, although different from it both in its proximate cause and in its treatment. Should we call this chronic state of dysentery diarrhea? Is it now inappropriate to administer purgatives?

I have no doubt that this chronic dysentery often, but not always, begins with looseness in the bowels. I have noticed many cases are the result of obstructions and the deathly condition in which the intestines are found, as the dissections have demonstrated. As much as the patient's strength is unable to support the action of the purgative, very mild laxatives must be applied. One spoonful of castor oil or some grains of rhubarb or ipecac[95] will provide the cure.

Opium cannot be dispensed for only one night in this chronic condition. It should be combined with the laxatives to make it more effective.

During the first attack of dysentery, when the bowel pains and tenesmus accompany the evacuation, astringents are the worst poison that can be given to the patient. Very few patients who take an astringent during the first attack will survive. The astringents will encourage spasms and can hinder other treatments. The lack of knowledge about the nature of the complaint is what has made some physicians resort to them and insist on their use. Indeed, it would be more humane to leave dysenteric patients untreated than to administer astringents to then.

However, when there are only frequent fluxes without either pain or tenesmus, then astringents can be beneficial. Although in this case the complaint cannot be called dysentery, but more correctly diarrhea. Dysentery can also become diarrhea, in which case it is more suitable to administer *catechu*, or *terra japonica* resin, extract of logwood, *quassia amara*, *simarouba*,[96] kino gum (the nutritious one), wine, etc.

Bloodletting has been recommended by some authors and condemned by others. The appearance of inflammation in the intestines has been determined by some to justify this evacuation. However, we must concede that many inflammations do not respond well to bloodletting, and dysentery is certainly among them. I have sometimes let blood, but I have never found it provides any benefit. I have since stopped making observations of this because I immediately administer a purgative in order not to lose any time, which with this illness is so very precious and short.

Essays on Tetanus in Angola

I define tetanus as the "spasmodic rigidity of the flexor muscles of the neck, the spine, and sometimes of the extremities, occasional convulsive shocks that cause seizures throughout the body, which are accompanied with violent pain, lockjaw, hardening of the bowels, and difficulty swallowing."

Most physicians, both ancient and modern, divide tetanus into several species.[97] It is called *opisthotonos* when the contractions in the muscles of the back and near the spine are so powerful that the head is pulled backward. It is called *emprosthotonos* when the muscles above the neck contract, pushing the head toward the chest. However, it seems to me that this distinction is inappropriate, given that the nature of the illness is always the same, and when the treatment does not differ. Such variations are not enough to describe different illnesses; rather, they only serve to introduce into medicine a large number of useless names that make it more difficult for those who wish to commit them to memory and serve to confuse the same maladies. As for the other types of tetanus, we also have lateral and pleurothotonic, both of which names are equally unnecessary. The *catocho* described by Sauvages[98] is not a different genus of tetanus just because it lacks symptoms of *dyspnea*.[99] In the same way we can also dismiss the divisions into tonic, holotonic, cervine, traumatic, etc., tetanus, and the need for particular treatments.

History of Tetanus

Tetanus can affect any person of any age and of either sex, though it affects adults more than children and only very rarely manifests in women. The early symptom is a slight stiffness in the neck that gradually increases until it becomes difficult to move the head, which then becomes sore. The stiffness soon moves into the tongue, making it difficult to swallow. It soon becomes impossible to move the neck, and the muscles begin to harden, particularly the sterno-mastoid. A violent shooting pain goes from the sternum to the back, and with that the body stiffens, causing it to arch; the jaws clench against the teeth, the belly rises, and there is a considerable swelling of the navel; the head is thrown backward, making it impossible for food to make its way to the stomach; breathing is quickened and the bowels are restricted.

All these symptoms increase, and the violent spasms extend to the extremities. The contractions become more frequent and are always accompanied by a sharp and intense pain that is relieved only when the muscles relax. However, this remission lasts only for a few minutes before it is swept away in a new contraction that comes without any evident cause. The pulse increases and becomes irregular; the face turns pale and is covered in a cold sweat. The unfortunate sufferer will remain in this condition for four or five days until a copious sweat befalls him until death frees the poor sufferer from such an intolerable torment and anguish.

Tetanus does not always strike with the violence described above. At times its symptoms are more gradual and progressive, while at yet others they suddenly manifest themselves in all their violence. In children I have seen it commence with continual tears and screams, without being able to find any cause whatsoever; they continually take and release their nursemaid's breast, and all efforts fail to induce them to suckle.

With some, the pulse remains regular; the body temperature normal; the head upright, but always rigid and immobile; the stomach flat, although always as hard as a board; the excretions sometimes change, while other times they remain perfect; sometimes the flow of urine stops, while at other times it flows normally, but always clear; sometimes the appetite remains, in others there is anorexia, although digestion is always good.

When the spasm passes into the extremities, the lower extremities almost always suffer the most. Sufferers are affected by a rigidity of such force that they find it physically impossible to bend their knees; their toes curve and are unable to straighten; the feet are bent almost in line with the shins. The arms are occasionally stricken with random spasms and remain able to move with ease while the rest of the body is completely immobile.

I have witnessed some in which the arms and legs are outstretched while the fingers and toes remain flexible and able to move. In other cases, this flexibility is partial, at times affecting only the fingers, then just the toes; at times all the toes in one foot, then some of the toes on the same foot or the same hand. I have also seen that occur during universal contractions: convulsions in the eyes, the forehead, the lips, the nose, and the ears, although such cases are rare. During contractions it is not uncommon for the patient to bare all his teeth, grimacing in absolute desperation.

After the illness has taken possession of the entire body, the slightest possible thing can provoke spasmodic contractions: if the patient tries to move himself, to speak, or even to swallow his own saliva, that is sufficient; it is even enough for the physician to touch the patient's arm in order to check his pulse for there to be an immediate convulsion.

Those patients who are stricken suddenly rarely survive, since the violence and severity of the spasm will not respond to remedies and will destroy the life force before any treatment has time to take effect. However, the attacks that come gradually give way to those remedies that are able to act, and fade away little by little as the treatment goes on. However, in gradual and violent attacks, should the patient survive the fourth day, he could well escape with his life, even when the symptoms appear grave. The convulsions never respond quickly, despite initially seeming that they will; rather, they slowly diminish in their force.

The deadly outcome of tetanus is always demonstrated in one of two ways: either the patient's body is covered in a profuse sweat or the extremities begin to chill, with the rest of the body retaining its natural temperature.

It has been known for a patient who has recovered from tetanus to be killed by a sudden despondency because of the despair that always remains. If this weakness is not caught in time by the physician or nurses, it will not in itself cost the life, although it will give time for the patient to be stricken by some of the diseases endemic to this country, and which will certainly lead to death. Such patients will normally succumb to coincident fevers and dysenteries.

If the fever strikes before the spasm has been eliminated, and within the four-day period during which the violent spasms normally end, it ordinarily leads to a favorable crisis that aids the selfsame spasms.* However, should this fever be accompanied by delirium, coma, or lethargy, it always ends badly. In such cases all the natural functions suffer, which with tetanus would normally remain unaffected. Dyspnea increases to the point that it causes total suffocation. The convulsions get stronger and more frequent. An extreme distress and mortal fatigue overwhelms all the senses, and death follows within a few hours.

The hardened bowels, a symptom of this malady from the outset, do not respond to purgatives, whether mild or powerful, so long as the spasms continue with strength. However, as soon as the spasms begin to fade, the bowels will relax to the same extent.

The reduction of the general spasm is recognized by the diminution of the trismus.[100] The head remains immobile and the neck remains stiff for many days after the patient is able to open his mouth and swallow food without difficulty. Flexibility later returns to the extremities and the other parts of the body until the patient is restored to his natural condition.

Proximate Cause

Since we entirely ignore the nature of muscular movements, we are not able to say what condition the muscles are in while in their rigid state, and therefore the proximate cause of tetanus remains obscure. The pathology of *simple solids*[101] cannot be properly separated from their physiology, and in this respect there has been little progress. Whatever Gaubius[102] wrote about solids, it is no more than the effects of causes he did not know, and which even now we ignore. Their prodigious nature in all their functions is never more admirable than in the voluntary movements we give our bodies. We imagine theories to explain this phenomenon, but how far from the truth are they? This is, however, the only means we have of getting close to it. Experiments, examinations, hypotheses: these are the only means of discovering that which

---

*A espasmo autem tetano detento febris superveniens solvit morbum. [When a fever occurs in a patient affected by spasms or tetanus, the malady is resolved.—Trans.] [See *Hippocratis Aphorismi*, 57:4.—Ed.]

the senses cannot reach. If no attempts are made—if human under-standing never emerges from the lethargy of the ignorance in which it was born—if these same systems that are now considered false and delusional had not been first, then science will not have changed, and it would be as it was when the world began. While the idea I propose may be a delusion, it will at least serve to provoke great minds to try to understand the error and to discover the truth. I will proceed to explain what I believe to be the proximate cause of tetanus.

Most writers who have approached this malady ignore the proxi-mate cause, perhaps fearing they will enter a chaos of difficulties and problems that are incomprehensible even today. Therefore, the treat-ment they prescribe, far from being established scientifically, is entirely empirical. Here I will seek to understand that cause, and where I am unable to discover the truth, I will at least seek to take us away from the old school sect that in centuries past hindered the progress of medicine and of which we should be ashamed to allow to appear in the present.

The solids in our body are divided into the simple and the vital: the former consist of the muscle mass, and the latter constitute a funda-mental part of the nerves. "Simple solids" [muscles] are found in both animate and inanimate bodies. Nerves ["vital solids"] are found only in animate bodies.

However, the simple solids in animate bodies, united with nerves by a cohesive force, enjoy a certain degree of flexibility and the elasticity necessary for animal functions. As soon as the vital solids lose that which animates and vivifies them, the simple solids will also lose their flexibility, as can be seen with cadavers. This flexibility has different degrees in the different parts of the body, that is to say, according to the particular nerves, or the different mix or organization of the solids.

These two properties of simple solids vary according to the condition and modification of the vital solids, to the atmospheric temperament to which the body is exposed, to the degree of extension they suffer, which is determined by the movements and respites to which they are accus-tomed, and according to the diseases they suffer. Herein is the reason that some corpses remain soft and flexible until the moment they are buried. Here we can also understand the reason why many solids are ossified when they should be naturally soft.

Simple solids can neither contract nor relax without the intervention of the vital solids with which they are united, just as in chemistry, when some bodies will not combine and others will not separate without a certain specific reactant agent.[103] When simple solids are separated from the vital solids, external causes will operate on them in the same way they operate on inanimate and mechanical bodies.

Therefore, the proximate cause of tetanus is the spasmodic contraction of the simple solids, which lose their flexibility by having received some influences from the vital solids.

That the spasm is in the "simple solids" and not the "vital solids" is proved by the following facts: regardless of how powerful the tetanus may be, the patient never loses his sensations as he would should the illness strike the nerves, as is the case with paralysis; with tetanus the patient always perspires, and at times he will sweat profusely, which should not happen if the nerves were attacked; with tetanus the natural functions do not experience much change, and as tetanus does not affect the brain, there is no delirium or confusion; this should be the case should the illness exist within the vital solids, that is, within the nervous system.

It is true that the first place the illness manifests is in the nerves, the sole principle, genesis, and cause of all of our body's actions. However, the same nerves, upon receiving sensations, communicate them to whichever parts of the body are receptive to them, from which follow a variety of diseases. Should it [the illness] come to the surface of the body it can produce spasms, the proximate cause of fevers and colds. It can enter the internal membranes and cause inflammations, and if it reaches the intestines it can lead to dysentery and other disorders common to this area. If it reaches the simple solids it will lead to tetanus.

The means by which contractions consequent to tetanus are produced remains unclear. The solution to the mystery raises only doubts and reminds us of our total ignorance. It is more the duty of the physiologist to seek to uncover this secret than it is the duty of the therapist or pathologist. For them, it is enough to know what causes the illness, while ignoring how these causes function in the system. We must be content with facts, for reason cannot discover more, and our reason is barred from seeking to know those things that are superior to us.

Remote Causes

The remote causes of tetanus are all of those that damage the nerves operating the muscles to such an extent and with such force that they cause lesions on the simple solids with which they are linked, and by means of which those simple solids function.

The causes of such damage to the nerves can be considered to be either generic or topical: the former strike the entire nervous system, while the latter strike only a part of it.

Generic causes include cold, dampness suddenly applied to a warm body, acute fevers, hysterical afflictions, and paralysis. Could syphilis also be a remote cause of tetanus, as some suggest? I believe there is no basis for responding yes.

Topical causes are wounds, ulcers, blows, contusions, fractures, dislocations, amputations, falls, or any other lesion on any part of the body. They can also be caused by worms that penetrate the intestines and burrow through to the abdominal cavity or remain suspended between the two. I have seen such things. I witnessed one patient die of tetanus because of a tooth extraction in which the dentist needed to make four strenuous attempts before the tooth came out. There are an infinite number of such examples.

It should be noted that when tetanus begins from these topical causes, the attack will not immediately cause damage to the nerves with lesions; rather, it will take days for this to manifest. However, when beginning from generic causes, the complaint manifests immediately and progresses rapidly.

Cure

Now I can boast that I have found an excellent method of treating tetanus, one that has always produced good results. More patients are cured than die since I have begun administering this treatment. It is very simple, and the remedies are the same as those exalted by Lind, Home, Laroche, Duboueix, Hillary, Chalmers, and others who have written on this infirmity. However, the advantage I have obtained over all of them, and the benefit this has had for mankind, was obtained by increasing the dose of the very same remedies to such a degree that it overcame the spasm, and by knowing how far one could go without endangering the patient.

The hot baths recommended by some, and the cold baths recommended by others, seem to me to be entirely useless, for in my experience they have never produced beneficial outcomes. Similarly, I consider the use of cold water in the more serious cases to be worthless, and so I absolutely refuse to apply it, preferring to use the time in the administration of other more decisive treatments in which I have faith. Caustics are similarly useless, and experience has led me to ignore these in similar complaints. There is no profit in using antispasmodics. I am not convinced, as Bajon believes, that they are inappropriate let alone harmful, but I believe their benefit is too small and limited to overcome such a powerful complaint. As we shall see, even the more effective remedies need to be administered in extraordinary doses before they have any effect.

Bloodletting is always harmful, even when the patient's constitution is plethoric and seems to indicate the need for it. If the appearance of the patient's blood serves to move the physician to deliberate over the necessity for bloodletting, the blood in tetanus seems to forbid him from tampering with it. We must avoid bloodletting in these illnesses accompanied by weakness, or for which such debility is a proximate cause. Tetanus is such an illness in which the life force is both weak and fading.

As soon as the patient appears to have been struck by tetanus, I will have the back, neck, and especially the thighs rubbed with a mercurial unguent.* I will follow this by making the patient drink a high dose of opium tincture† to ensure he has rest. If six hours pass during which the patient does not sleep, I will give him a double dose of opium, which will normally enable him to sleep for a few minutes. The next day I will have his body rubbed again with the mercurial unguent; and in the morning will administer one hundred drops of opium tincture, and the same again in the afternoon. I will repeat the application of the

---

*Mercurial unguent, one ounce.
†Opium tincture, 100 drops; mixed with musk, two ounces: stir.

unguent on the third day, but with only half the dose of the previous day, and will continue to administer the same dosage of opium tincture.

Ptyalism[104] will appear during the course of the fourth day, which is when I will suspend the application of mercurial rubs. At this point I will continue to administer opium in the morning and afternoon until the trismus has gone and the tongue is able to move.

Should there be no more incidents, I believe the patient to be out of danger the moment the ptyalism manifests, and there is therefore no need for the doses of opium to be so high. Once the trismus has been overcome I will suspend the morning dose but retain that given in the afternoon. I will then reduce this dose by ten drops each day until the dosage is twenty drops, which I will continue to administer until the patient has been restored.

Since with tetanus the throat is usually blocked, it is often necessary to introduce the opium in an enema. In such cases both the morning and afternoon doses should be double that taken by mouth.* Soups should also be introduced in the same way in order to keep the patient alive. However, opium is normally retained in one way or the other by the natural constriction that always persists in the bowels.

As soon as the violence of both the trismus and the overall spasm diminishes, care should be taken to free the bowels, which will now respond to treatment. On this occasion a purgative will help nature remove the spasm, while at the same time reducing the ptyalism that was a side effect of the mercury applied at the height of the illness.

Some mistakenly believe it takes days for the mercury to have an effect in the system. Their argument that the ptyalism manifests only some time after the application of the mercury does not prove it takes time to have an effect, but rather it shows the dose is limited so that it does not produce saliva quickly. How often has a purgative containing mercury been administered, only for us to find on the following day the patient who took it with his tongue and face swollen, his teeth loose, and spitting profusely? Everything depends on the dose and on the disposition of nature.

*Opium tincture, 200 drops. Chicken broth, enough for an enema: mix together.

After the patient has evacuated his bowels and is completely clear of tetanus, I will begin administrating tonics to restore strength. My preferred tonic is Peruvian bark, and I administer one-eighth ounce to the patient each day. I also prescribe wine, which invigorates the system and helps prevent another illness from striking a recovering body that is susceptible to illness.

When there are no violent symptoms with the tetanus, the patient can often be cured by administering a small dose of opium each hour until he falls asleep. However, this method is too gentle and will not help when the tetanus is accompanied by trismus and other serious symptoms, because there will never be enough opium in the stomach to provide relief since the proportions introduced through an hourly dose of opium will have little effect as the benefits of the first doses begin to wear off.

If the tetanus is topical, the treatment can be abbreviated by making a deep incision above the lesion in order to cut the nerves and break the communication. The patient will feel immediate relief, and nature will overcome the spasms. However, I always assist nature in these cases, so that the illness can be more easily removed.

THE END

Notes

1. This was the highest medical office in the colony; Azeredo's posting placed him effectively in charge of all medical services in Angola. — Ed.

2. The most prevalent fever in this zone was malaria, and it is almost certainly to this illness that the author most frequently refers; however, several other maladies existed that fell within the general term "fevers," and these are also addressed here. — Trans.

3. Sir John Pringle (1707–82), Scottish physician with noted expertise in military medicine. It appears that here Azeredo wishes to confirm his knowledge of contemporary medical authors who had written on the symptoms, causes, and treatment of fevers. — Ed.

4. James Lind (1716–94), Scottish physician who experimented with cures for scurvy. — Ed.

5. George Cleghorn (1716–94), Scottish physician who helped disseminate knowl-

edge of cinchona, also known as "Peruvian bark" (the source of quinine) as a cure for malaria and other fevers. — Ed.

6. James Badenoch (active c. 1770), Scottish physician known for his work on methods to treat scurvy at sea. — Ed.

7. John Clark (1744–1805), Scottish physician known for his work on the treatment of diseases common on long sea voyages in the tropics, and his advocacy of the application of quinine-containing Peruvian bark for fevers. — Ed.

8. This is most likely a reference to Gilbert Blane (1749–1832), a Scottish physician who instituted health reform in the Royal Navy to eliminate scurvy among sailors. — Ed.

9. John Hunter (1728–93), Scottish surgeon and advocate of the scientific method. — Ed.

10. Thomas Sydenham (1624–89), English physician known as the "English Hippocrates." — Ed.

11. Azeredo here uses the clinical word "affection," taken from the Latin *afectio*, which is the term William Cullen used. The word encompasses a wide range of semantic meanings; for example, it could be translated variously as inflammation, infection, disorder, or distemper, among other terms. — Ed.

12. *Phlegmasia* was a generic term for inflammation; modern researchers have associated this malady with a severe form of deep venous thrombosis, which results from extensive blockage of the major and branching veins in the arms or legs. — Ed.

13. An abnormal elevation of body temperature; that is, fever. — Ed.

14. *Phlogistic*: of or relating to inflammations and fevers. *Diathesis*: a tendency to suffer from a particular medical condition. Thus, a tendency to suffer from fevers or inflammations. — Ed.

15. *Synochus*: a continuous fever; unabated pyrexia. — Ed.

16. *Idiopathic*: a disease apparently arising spontaneously, or from an obscure or unknown cause; a disorder for which the cause may not be readily apparent or characterized. — Ed.

17. Azeredo mentions, somewhat arbitrarily, many contemporary names for fevers, the terms for which are often Latin based; some of these he borrowed from William Cullen's text (1780, vol. 2). — Ed.

18. Francis Bacon, First Viscount of St. Albans (1561–1626), English statesman and pioneer of the scientific method. — Ed.

19. Here Azeredo takes his description of attacks and symptoms of fevers from William Cullen, *First Lines of the Practice of Physic*, 4 vols. (Edinburgh, 1784), vol. 1, p. 10. — Ed.

20. Sixteenth-century medical term meaning to be suffering from *cachexia*, a state of general physical wasting and malnutrition, associated with suffering from a chronic disease. See below. — Ed.

21. That is, *edema*: an abnormal infiltration and excess accumulation of serous fluid in connective tissue or in a serous cavity. — Ed.

22. General ill health with emaciation, usually occurring in association with cancer or a chronic infectious disease. See Ephraim Chambers, *Cyclopaedia, or, an Universal Dictionary of Arts and Sciences*, 2 vols. (London, 1728), which defines *cachexia*

as "an ill habit or disposition of body wherein the nutrition is depraved throughout the whole habit, at once, frequently leading towards a dropsy."—Ed.

23. Regarding the use of quinine (also known as "Jesuit's" or "Peruvian" Bark) see Cullen (1784), §212, p. 188, and (1789), vol. 2, pp. 53, 89.—Ed.

24. *Petechiae* are symptomatic marks or blemishes on the skin caused by fever or other disease.—Ed.

25. Azeredo's reference is to the eighteenth-century concept of "crisis," meaning the crucial turning point of a disease. See Théophile de Bordeu, "Crise," in Denis Diderot and Jean Le Rond d'Alembert, eds., *Encyclopédie ou dictionnaire raisonné des sciences, des arts et des métiers*, 28 vols. (Paris, 1751–72), vol. 4 (1754), pp. 471–89.—Ed.

26. Asclepiades of Bithynia (c. 124–40 BCE), critic of Hippocrates's humoral doctrine.—Ed.

27. Themison of Laodicea (c. first century BCE), Greek physician and founder of the methodic school of medicine.—Ed.

28. Aulus Cornelius Celsus (c. 25 BCE–50 CE), Roman encyclopedist.—Ed.

29. Aelius Galenus (Galen) (Pergamon, c. 129–216 CE), Roman physician.—Ed.

30. That is, Philippus Aureolus Theophrastus Bombastus von Hohenheim (c. 1493–1541), Swiss physician, alchemist, and botanist.—Ed.

31. William Harvey (1578–1657), English physician who first comprehensively described blood, the heart, and the circulatory system.—Ed.

32. Gjuro (Georgius) Baglivi (Dubrovnik, 1668–1707), Italian physician who advanced the theory that the solid parts of organs are more crucial to their good functioning than their fluids.—Ed.

33. A "lentor" is a distinct diagnostic concept developed by the Dutch physician Herman Boerhaave; it connotes a theoretical viscous abnormal bodily fluid thought to be related to the genesis of fevers.—Ed.

34. "Pitkarn" in the original. Archibald Pitcairn (1652–1713), Scottish physician who taught medicine at Leiden, once was erroneously believed to have instructed Boerhaave.—Ed.

35. Giovanni Alfonso Borelli (Naples, 1608–79), Italian biomechanist, physiologist, and mathematician.—Ed.

36. Nicolas Lémery (1645–1715), French chemist.—Trans.

37. Herman Boerhaave (1668–1738), Dutch botanist and physician who pioneered clinical teaching and diagnostic medicine.—Ed.

38. William Hewson (1739–1774), English surgeon, physiologist, and anatomist; known for early studies of hematology.—Ed.

39. Friedrich Hoffman (Halle, 1660–1742), German physician who championed the study of the nervous system.—Ed.

40. Albrecht von Haller (1708–77), Swiss anatomist.—Ed.

41. Robert Whytt (1714–66), Scottish physician and professor of medicine at Edinburgh University.—Ed.

42. Hieronymus David Gaubius (Heidelberg, 1705–80), German physician and chemist.—Ed.

43. Thomas Willis (1621–75), English physician and founding member of the Royal Society.—Ed.

44. John Brown (1735–88), Scottish physician who published *Elementa medicinae* (1780).—Ed.

45. "Animal economy" was a very precise physiological and medical concept during the Enlightenment; the idea marked a departure from the old vision of the living creature being composed of a body and a soul, and from the Hippocratic corporeal humoristic tradition in medicine. See Philippe Huneman, "'Animal Economy': Anthropology and the Rise of Psychiatry from the *Encyclopédie* to the Alienists," in *The Anthropology of the Enlightenment*, ed. Larry Wolff and Marco Cipolloni (Stanford, CA: Stanford University Press, 2007), pp. 262–76.—Ed.

46. Tenesmus: a straining urge to urinate or defecate, without the ability to do so. —Ed.

47. Azeredo's precise term was *disponent causes.*—Ed.

48. For a description of the contemporary city of Luanda see A. Magno de Castilho, *Descripção e roteiro da costa occidental de África: Desde o cabo de Espartel até o das Agulhas*, 2 vols. (Lisbon: Imprensa Nacional, 1866), vol. 2, p. 209; and Ilídio Amaral, *Luanda: Estudo de geografia urbana* (Lisbon: Tipografia Atlântida Editora, 1968), p. 42. —Ed.

49. Jan Ingenhousz (1730–99), Dutch physiologist, biologist, and chemist who discovered photosynthesis.—Ed.

50. Note Azeredo's explanation of "mephitic air" (also referred to by the French term *azote*) in his "Chemical Examination of the Atmosphere of Rio de Janeiro" in *Jornal Encyclopédico* (Lisbon: Officina de Antonio Rodrigues Galhardo, March 1790), p. 264.—Ed.

51. *Euphorbia tirucalli.*—Trans.

52. *Massangralá*, in the original, also known as sorghum.—Ed.

53. From the coco family of plants.—Trans.

54. Bean pods.—Trans.

55. *Aloe littoralis.*—Trans.

56. Karaya gum tree.—Trans.

57. A genus of the Phyllanthaceae family of plant.—Trans.

58. *Cassia occidentalis.*—Trans.

59. *siliqua* in the original; that is, a fruit consisting of two dehiscent pods or capsules.—Ed.

60. Indian spurge tree (*Euphorbia tirucalli*).—Trans.

61. *Quibungo* in the original.—Ed. This may be a mistake or typographical error for *quibondo*, which is the wild African tragacanth tree (*Sterculia tragacantha*). —Trans.

62. The *Ficus thonningii*, or bark-cloth fig tree. In Kimbundu, one of the main languages of Angola, this tree was called *nzanda* (thus the phonetic Portuguese name *Insandeira*) and was a symbol of royalty in Angola.—Ed.

63. The disease scurvy, now understood to be the result of vitamin deficiency, was known in contemporary vernacular Portuguese as the *mal de Luanda* (that is, the disease or malady of Luanda). Regarding the "malady of Luanda" see Aleixo de Abreu (1568–1630), *Tratado de las siete enfermedades: De la inflammacion vniuersal del Higado, Zirbo, Pyloron, y Riñones, y de la obstrucion, de la satiriasi, de la terciana y febre maligna,*

y passion hipocondriaca: Lleua otros tres tratados, del mal de Loanda, del Guzano, y de las Fuentes y Sedales. . . . (Lisbon, Pedro Craesbeeck, 1623). — Ed.

64. *Carneirada* literally means a carnage or butchery, but it was the common name in Portuguese colonies in coastal Africa for a class of seasonal illnesses, broadly associated with bouts or epidemics of malaria. See Rafael Bluteau, *Vocabulario portuguez e latino* . . . , 10 vols. (Coimbra: Collegio das Artes da Companhia de Jesu, 1712–28), vol. 2, p. 153; and António Houaiss (director), Mauro de Salles Villar, and Francisco Manoel de Mello Franco, *Dicionário Houaiss da língua portuguesa*, 3 vols. (Lisbon: Círculo de Leitores, 1999–2003), pp. 816, 2356. — Ed.

65. Azeredo here used the specific term *mephitic gas*, now known as carbon dioxide. For comparison see Azeredo, "Exame quimico da atmosphera do Rio de Janeiro," *Jornal Encyclopédico* (Lisbon: Officina de Antonio Rodrigues Galhardo, March 1790), p. 264. — Ed.

66. For comparison see António Ribeiro Sanches, *Tratado da conservação da saúde dos povos: Obra util e igualmente necessaria a os magistrados, capitaens generais, capitaens de mar, e guerra, prelados, abadessas, médicos, e pays de familia.* . . . (Paris, 1756). — Ed.

67. Azeredo here refers to Isaac Maddox, *The Expediency of Preventive Wisdom: A Sermon Preached before the Right Honourable the Lord-Mayor, the Aldermen, and Governors of Several Hospitals of the City of London. At St Bridget's Church, on Easter-Monday, 1750.* . . . (London: H. Woodfall, 1751). — Ed.

68. In the original, *Amendubís.* — Ed.

69. *Água de Inglaterra* (English tonic water): general name for a prepared patent medicine composed of tonic water and a quinine infusion, first marketed in the late seventeenth century by Fernando Mendes (1645?–1724), an expatriate Portuguese *converso* physician living in London. — Ed.

70. Azeredo's original phrase here, *bálsamo católico,* or "catholic balsam," refers to a prepared medicinal balm, usually composed with tincture of benzoin. See *Pharmacopeia Geral*, vol. 2, p. 208. — Ed.

71. Named after its inventor, the English physician Robert James (1703–76). — Trans.

72. Caustic: a medical substance applied topically to cause a burning or stinging sensation, or as an escharotic or corrosive agent to living tissue. — Ed.

73. During the Enlightenment, the medical term "quotidian" connoted (as it still does) a quite precise type of fever (the fit having an interval of twenty-four hours). See Cullen (1827), vol. 1, pp. 487, 538. — Ed.

74. *Tertian* and *quartian* fevers: precise contemporary medical terms meaning fevers with, respectively, a duration of forty-eight and seventy-two hours. See Cullen (1827), vol. 1, pp. 487, 535. — Ed.

75. See Cullen (1780), vol. 2, p. 171; and (1784), vol. 3, pp. 81, 101. — Ed.

76. Sir George Baker (1722–1809), English physician. — Trans.

77. In the original, *monco.* — Ed.

78. Small round nodules. See John Pringle, *Observations on Diseases of the Army* (London, 1775), p. 248. — Ed.

79. Cachexic: a physical state demonstrating general ill health with emaciation, usually occurring in association with a chronic debilitating disease. — Ed.

80. Scybala: hardened, semi-spherical masses of feces.—Ed.

81. Sanies: a thin, often greenish serous fluid that is discharged from ulcers, wounds, or abrasions.—Ed.

82. Sebaceous: fatty, greasy; of the nature of or resembling tallow or fat.—Ed.

83. See John Pringle, *Observations on Diseases of the Army* (London, 1775), p. 229. This is an early description of adipose tissue.—Ed.

84. Thomas Bartholin (1616–80), Danish physician best known for his work in the discovery of the lymphatic system in humans.—Ed.

85. Carl Linnaeus (1707–78), Swedish physician best known for the modern system of binomial botanical nomenclature. Azeredo's reference here seems to have been taken from Pringle, *Observations on Diseases of the Army*, p. 256.—Ed.

86. Azeredo's reference here seems to have been taken from Pringle, *Observations on Diseases of the Army*, p. 239.—Ed.

87. Omentum: a fold of the peritoneum connecting the stomach and the abdominal viscera, forming a protective and supporting covering membrane.—Ed.

88. Mesentery: the membrane that attaches the intestines to the posterior wall of the abdomen, holding them in position within the abdominal cavity, and supplying them with blood vessels, nerves, and lymphatics.—Ed.

89. Villous: covered or furnished with *villi*; that is, having small hairs.—Ed.

90. Ileum: the third and lowest division of the small intestine.—Ed.

91. Giovanni Battista Morgagni (1682–1771), Italian anatomist who championed anatomical pathology.—Ed.

92. Ipecacuanha: a flowering plant found mainly in Brazil and Peru, the root of which was made into medicines; its use was as an emetic or purgative. Ipecacuanha is the key ingredient in modern syrup of ipecac, used to induce vomiting.—Ed.

93. Cantharides tincture: solution made of alcohol and Spanish fly, an insect with, historically, multiple apothecary applications.—Ed.

94. Vesicatoria: Azeredo here refers to a caustic blistering agent derived from a type of beetle, *Lytta vesicatoria*, popularly referred to as "Spanish fly," that is common in southern Europe and central Asia. The substance, called a "cantharide," has been used in a range of medicinal applications from ancient times until the present day.—Ed.

95. *Cipó* and ipecacuanha (ipecac) were sometimes used interchangeably in eighteenth-century Portuguese and Brazilian medical texts.—Ed.

96. Plant of the Burseraceae family.—Trans.

97. See Cullen (1780), vol. 2, p. 209; and (1784), vol. 3, p. 282.—Ed.

98. François Boissier de Sauvages de Lacroix (1706–67), French physician. "Catocho" is the trancelike phase of catalepsy in which the patient is conscious but cannot move or speak; see Sauvages de Lacroix, *Nosologia methodica sistens morborum classes genera et species juxta sydenhami mentem et botanicorum ordinem*, 5 vols. (Amsterdam: De Tournes, 1763), vol. 2, p. 34; and Sauvages de Lacroix, *Nosologie methodique, dans laquelle les maladies sont rangées par classes, suivant le systême de Sydenham, & l'ordre des botanistes*, 3 vols. (Paris: Hérissant, 1770–71), vol. 1, p. 738.—Ed.

99. Dyspnea: difficult or labored breathing.—Ed.

100. Trismus: a spasm of the jaw muscles that makes opening the mouth difficult; lockjaw.—Ed.

101. That is, muscles. Azeredo refers to a precise concept used by Cullen to refer to muscle mass. See *Works* (1827), vol. 1, p. 10.—Ed.

102. Hieronymus David Gaubius (1705–80), German physician and author of *Institutiones pathologiae medicinalis* (1758).—Trans.

103. Modern science would call a reactant agent a "catalyst," but that term was not coined until 1794, and was not in general use before approximately 1835.—Ed.

104. Ptyalism: excessive secretion of saliva.—Ed.

BIBLIOGRAPHY

Primary Sources and Contemporary Works
(including those cited by Azeredo)

Abreu, Aleixo de. *Tratado de las siete enfermedades: De la inflammacion vniuersal del higado, zirbo, pyloron, y riñones, y de la obstrucion, de la satiriasi, de la terciana y febre maligna, y passion hipocondriaca: Lleua otros tres tratados, del mal de Loanda, del Guzano, y de las Fuentes y Sedales.* . . . Lisbon: Pedro Craesbeeck, 1623.

Anonymous. *Pharmacopeia Geral para o Reino e Domínios de Portugal.* . . . 2 vols. Lisbon: Regia Officina Typografica, 1794.

Azeredo, José Pinto de. *Ensaios sobre algumas enfermidades de Angola.* Lisbon: Régia Oficina Tipográfica, 1799.

———. "Exame quimico da atmosphera do Rio de Janeiro." In *Jornal Encyclopédico dedicado á Rainha N. Senhora, e destinado para instrucção geral com a notícia dos novos descobrimentos em todas as sciencias, e artes,* pp. 259–88. Lisbon: Oficina de António Rodrigues Galhardo, March 1790.

———. "Isagòge pathologica do corpo humano dedicada a Sua Alteza Real o Principe Regente Nosso Senhor." Manuscript, dated 1802. Biblioteca Nacional de Portugal, *códice* 8482.

———. "Oração de Sapiência feita e recitada no dia 11 de Setembro de 1791." Manuscript, 1791. Biblioteca Nacional de Portugal, *códice* 8486, ff. 1–7v.

Badenoch, James. "Observations on the Bilious Fever Usual in Voyages to the East Indies." In *Medical Observations and Inquiries by a Society of Physicians in London,* vol. 4, pp. 156–67. London: T. Cadell, 1771.

———. "Observations on the Use of Wort in the Cure of the Scurvy at Sea." In *Medical Observations and Inquiries by a Society of Physicians in London,* vol. 5, pp. 61–72. London: T. Cadell, 1776.

Blane, Gilbert. *Observations on the Diseases Incident to Seamen.* London: J. Cooper, 1785.

Boerhaave, Herman. *Dr. Boerhaave's Academical Lectures on the Theory of Physic: Being a Genuine Translation of His Institutes and Explanatory Comment.* . . . 6 vols. London: W. Innys, 1742–49.

Clark, John. *Observations on the Diseases in Long Voyages to Hot Countries, and Particularly on Those Which Prevail in the East Indies.* London: D. Wilson and G. Nicol, 1773.

Cullen, William. *First Lines of the Practice of Physics.* 4th ed., corrected and enlarged. 4 vols. Edinburgh: C. Elliot and T. Cadell, 1784.

———. *Institutions of Medicine. Part I. Physiology. For the Use of the Students in the University of Edinburgh.* 3rd ed. Edinburgh: Charles Elliot and T. Cadwell, 1785.

Bibliography

————. *Synopsis nosologiae methodicae, exhibens clariss. virorum Sauvagesii, Linnaei, Vogelii, et Sagari, systemata nosologica. Edidit suumque proprium systema nosologicum adjecit Gulielmus Cullen.* . . . 3rd ed. 2 vols. Edinburgh: William Creech, 1780; and London: T. Cadell & J. Murray, 1780.

————. *A Treatise of the Materia Medica.* 2 vols. Edinburgh: Charles Elliot, 1789, and London: C. Elliot & T. Kay, 1789.

————. *The Works of William Cullen, M.D.* . . . *Containing His Physiology, Nosology, and First Lines of the Practice of Physic: With Numerous Extracts from His Manuscript Papers, and from His Treatise of the Materia Medica.* 2 vols. Edited by John Thomson. Edinburgh: William Blackwood, 1827, and London: T. & G. Underwood, 1827.

Fontana, Felix. "Experiments and Observations on the Inflammable Air Breathed by Various Animals." *Philosophical Transactions of the Royal Society of London* 69 (1779): pp. 337–61.

Gilchrist, Ebenezer. *The Use of Sea Voyages in Medicine.* Appendix: "Concerning Bathing in Fevers." London: A. Millar, D. Wilson and T. Durham, 1756.

Henriques, Francisco da Fonseca. *Medicina lusitana: Socorro delphico, aos clamores da natureza humana, para total profligação de seus males.* . . . 2nd ed. Amsterdam: Miguel Diaz, 1731.

Hippocrates, Lucas Verhoofd, Theodoor Jansson ab Almeloveen, Aulus Cornelius Celsus, Herman Boerhaave, and Anne-Charles Lorry. *Hippocratis Aphorismi: Hippocratis et Celsi locis parallelis illustrati, studio et curâ Janssonii ab Almeloveen, D.M.* . . . Paris: apud Theophilum Barrois juniorem, 1784.

Hunter, John. *Observations on the Diseases of the Army in Jamaica; and on the Best Means of Preserving the Health of Europeans in That Climate.* London: G. Nicol, 1788.

Jackson, Robert. *A Treatise on the Fevers of Jamaica: With Some Observations on the Intermitting Fever of America, and an Appendix, Containing Some Hints on the Means of Preserving the Health of Soldiers in Hot Climates.* London: J. Murray, 1791.

Nabuco, Manuel Fernandes. "Observaçoens medico-chi[r]urgicas, anatomicas: Unicas até os nossos tempos, nas quaes se demonstra até onde tenho chegado com adossis [*sic*] do opio tebaico, em substancia; e laudano liquido, para serem assistidas as contracçoens convulsivas rezultadas das feridas, e chagas mais acontecimentos ofensivos e poderem de hoje em diante servir de guia no exercicio curatorio aos professores da Medicina Cirurgical." Manuscript, Bahia, Brazil, dated 15 November 1785. 189 pages. Biblioteca Nacional de Portugal, *códice* 11241.

————. *Observações médico-cirurgicas e anatómicas.* . . . Edited by Augusto Silva Carvalho. Porto: Tipográfia Domingos d'Oliveira, 1949.

Pringle, John. "A Continuation of the Experiments on Substances Resisting Putrefaction." *Philosophical Transactions of the Royal Society of London* 46 (1749–50): pp. 525–34.

————. "Further Experiments on Substances Resisting Putrefaction; With Experiments upon the Means of Hastening and Promoting It." *Philosophical Transactions of the Royal Society of London* 46 (1749–50): pp. 550–58.

Bibliography

————. *Observations on the Diseases of the Army*. 7th ed., revised and corrected. London: W. Strahan, [. . .] T. Durham, and T. Cadell, 1775.

————. "Some Experiments on Substances Resisting Putrefaction." *Philosophical Transactions of the Royal Society of London* 46 (1749–50): pp. 480–88.

Priestley, Joseph. *Directions for Impregnating Water with Fixed Air: In Order to Communicate to It the Peculiar Spirit and Virtues of Pyrmont Water, and Other Mineral Waters of a Similar Nature*. London: J. Johnson, 1772.

Robertson, Robert. *A Physical Journal Kept on Board His Majesty's Ship* Rainbow, *during Three Voyages to the Coast of Africa and West Indies, in the Year 1772, 1773, and 1774: To Which Is Prefixed, a Particular Account of the Remitting Fever, Which Happened on Board of His Majesty's Sloop* Weasel, *on That Coast, in 1769*. London: E. and C. Dilly, 1777.

Rosa, João Ferreira da. *Tratado único da constituição pestilencial de Pernambuco*. . . . Lisbon: Officina Miguel Menescal, 1694.

Royal College of Physicians, London. *Pharmacopoeia Collegii Regalis Medicorum Londinensis*. London: apud Josephum Johnson, 1788.

Sauvages de Lacroix, François Boissier de. *Nosologia methodica sistens morborum classes genera et species juxta sydenhami mentem et botanicorum ordinem*. 5 vols. Amsterdam: De Tournes, 1763.

————. *Nosologie methodique, dans laquelle les maladies sont rangées par classes, suivant le systême de Sydenham, & l'ordre des botanistes*. 3 vols. Paris: Hérissant, 1770–71.

Semedo, João Corvo. *Polyanthea medicinal: Noticias galenicas, e chymicas, repartidas em tres tratados, dedicadas . . . Cardeal de Sousa, Arcebispo de Lisboa*. . . . 3rd ed., revised and expanded. Lisbon: Officina de Antonio Pedrozo Galram, 1716.

Stahl, Georg Ernst. *Theoria medica vera: Physiologiam et pathologiam; Tanquam doctrinae medicae partes*. . . . Halle: Typis et Impensis Orphanotrophei, 1706–8.

Secondary Sources and Reference Works

SECONDARY SOURCES

Amaral, Ilídio. *Luanda: Estudo de geografia urbana*. Lisbon: Tipografia Atlântida editora, 1968.

Breyner, Francisco de Melo (Fourth Conde de Ficalho). *Plantas úteis da África portuguesa*. 2nd ed., revised and with a new preface by Ruy Telles Palhinha. Lisbon: Agência Geral das Colonias, 1947.

Bynum, William F., and Vivian Nutton, eds. *Theories of Fever from Antiquity to the Enlightenment*. Vol. 1 of *Medical History:* supplement. London: Wellcome Institute for the History of Medicine Medical History, 1981.

Castilho, A. Magno de. *Descripção e roteiro da costa occidental de Africa: Desde o cabo de Espartel até o das Agulhas*. 2 vols. Lisbon: Imprensa Nacional, 1866.

Chodos, Marc. "Sir John Pringle: The Neglected Eighteenth-Century Environmentalist." Los Angeles: UCLA School of Medicine, 1996.

DeLacy, Margaret E. "A Linnaean Thesis Concerning *Contagium Vivum*: The

Bibliography

'Exanthemata Viva' of John Nyander and Its Place in Contemporary Thought, with a New Translation by A. J. Cain." *Medical History* 39 (1995): pp. 159–85.

Dias, José Pedro Sousa, and João Rui Rocha Pita. "L'influence de la pharmacie et de la chimie françaises au Portugal au XVIIIe siècle: Nicolas Lémery." *Revue d'Histoire de la Pharmacie* 82:300 (1994): pp. 84–90.

Franco, Odair. *História da febre-amarela no Brasil.* Rio de Janeiro: Ministério da Saúde, Departamento Nacional de Endemias Rurais, 1969.

Geggus, David. "Yellow Fever in the 1790s: The British Army in Occupied Saint Domingue." *Medical History* 23 (1979): pp. 38–58.

Gossweiler, John. *Flora exótica de Angola: Nomes vulgares e origem das plantas cultivadas ou sub-espontaneas.* Luanda: Imprensa Nacional, 1950. Offprint of Agronomia Angolana.

Haycock, David Boyd. "Exterminated by the Bloody Flux: Dysentery in Eighteenth-Century Naval and Military Medical Accounts." *Journal for Maritime Research* 4:1 (2002): pp. 15–39.

Johnstone, R. W. "William Cullen." *Medical History* 3 (1959): pp. 33–46.

Marques, Manuel Silvério, and António Braz de Oliveira. "José Pinto de Azeredo: A Cosmopolitan Physician from Rio. Revisiting His *Ensaios sobre algumas enfermidades de Angola.*" In *Percursos na história do livro médico (1450–1800)*, ed. Palmira Fontes da Costa and Adelino Cardoso, pp. 231–54. Lisbon: Edições Colibri, 2011.

Pinto, Manuel Serrano, Marco António Cecchini, Isabel Maria Malaquias, Lycia Maria Moreira-Nordemann, and João Rui Rocha Pita. "O medico brasileiro José Pinto de Azeredo (1766?–1810) e o exame químico da atmosfera do Rio de Janeiro." In *Manguinhos: História, Ciências, Saúde* 12:3 (September–December 2005): pp. 617–26.

Pita, João Rui Rocha. "Um livro com 200 anos: A farmacopeia portuguesa (edição oficial). A publicação da primeira farmacopeia oficial, *Pharmacopeia Geral* (1794)." *Revista de História das Ideias* 20 (1999): pp. 47–100.

Selwyn, Sydney. "Sir John Pringle: Hospital Reformer, Moral Philosopher and Pioneer of Antiseptics." *Medical History* 10:3 (July 1966): pp. 266–74.

Serrano, Eduardo. "Évolution et histoire de la pharmacie au Portugal." *Revue d'Histoire de la Pharmacie* 84:312 (1996): pp. 227–33.

Stott, Rosalie. "Health and Virtue: Or, How to Keep Out of Harm's Way; Lectures on Pathology and Therapeutics by William Cullen, c. 1770." *Medical History* 31:2 (1987): pp. 123–42.

Taylor, Georgette. "Unification Achieved: William Cullen's Theory of Heat and Phlogiston as an Example of His Philosophical Chemistry." *British Journal for the History of Science* 39:4 (2006): pp. 477–501.

Toledo Curbelo, Gabriel José. "La otra historia de la fiebre amarilla en Cuba: 1492–1909." *Revista Cubana de Higiene y Epidemiologia* 38:3 (October 2000): pp. 220–27.

Bibliography

REFERENCE WORKS

Assis Júnior, António de. *Dicionário Kimbundo-Português linguístico, botânico, histórico e corográfico, seguido de um índice alfabético dos nomes próprios.* Luanda: Argente, Santos & Companhia, 1941.

Bayle, Antoine L. Jessé, Auguste M. Thillaye, Daniel Leclerc, and Nicolas François Joseph Éloy. *Biographie médicale par ordre chronologique d'après Daniel Leclerc, Éloy, etc.* . . . 2 vols. Amsterdam: N. V. Boekhandel & Antiquariaat B. M. Israel, 1967.

Bluteau, Rafael. *Vocabulario portuguez e latino, aulico, anatomico, architectonico, bellico, botanico, brasilico, comico, critico, chimico, dogmatico, dialectico, dendrologico, ecclesiastico, etymologico, economico, florifero, forense, fructifero.* . . . 10 vols. Coimbra: Collegio das Artes da Companhia de Jesu, 1712–28.

Chambers, Ephraim. *Cyclopaedia, or, an Universal Dictionary of Arts and Sciences: Containing the Definitions of the Terms, and Accounts of the Things Signify'd Thereby, in the Several Arts, Both Liberal and Mechanical, and the Several Sciences, Human and Divine.* . . . 2 vols. London: James and John Knapton, et al., 1728.

Col de Villars, Élie. *Dictionnaire françois-latin, des termes de médecine, et de chirurgie, avec leur définition, leur division, & leur etymologie . . . Suite du cours de chirurgie.* Paris: Chez Le Mercier . . . et Herissant . . . , 1760.

Cunha, António Geraldo da, and António Houaiss, eds. *Dicionário histórico das palavras portuguesas de origem Tupi.* 2nd ed. São Paulo: Melhoramentos, 1982.

Dezeimeris, Jean-Eugène, Charles Prosper Ollivier, and Jacques Raige-Delorme. *Dictionnaire historique de la médecine ancienne et moderne, ou précis de l'histoire générale, technologique et littéraire de la médecine; suivi de la bibliographie médicale du dix-neuvième siècle; et d'un répertoire bibliographique par ordre de matières.* 4 vols. Paris: Béchet Jeune, 1828–39.

Fernandes, Rosette Batarda. "Glossário de termos botânicos." *Anuário da Sociedade Broteriana* 38 (1972): pp. 181–292. Revised and updated online edition by Fátima Sales (2007): http://www.uc.pt/herbario_digital/glossario/.

Houaiss, António (director), Mauro de Salles Villar, and Francisco Manoel de Mello Franco; Instituto Antônio Houaiss de Lexicografia. *Dicionário Houaiss da língua portuguesa.* 3 vols. Lisbon: Círculo de Leitores, 1999–2003.

Littré, Émile, and Charles Robin, eds. *Dictionnaire de médecine, de chirurgie, de pharmacie, de l'art vétérinaire et des sciences qui s'y rapportent.* 14th ed. Paris: J. B. Baillière et Fils, 1978.

Machado, José Pedro. *Grande dicionário da língua portuguesa.* Annotated by Fernando Sylvan. 2nd ed. 13 vols. Lisbon: Sociedade de Língua Portuguesa; Amigos do Livro, 1981–86.

Macquer, Pierre-Joseph. *Dictionnaire de chimie, contenant la théorie et la pratique de cette science, son application a la physique, a l'histoire naturelle.* . . . 2 vols. Paris: Chez Théophile Barrois, Libraire, 1778.

Quincy, John. *Lexicon Physico-Medicum, or New Medical Dictionary Explaining the Difficult Terms Used in the Several Branches of the Profession and in Such Parts of*

Bibliography

Natural Philosophy as Are Introductory Thereto. . . . 5th ed. London: T. Longman, 1736.

Valdez, Manuel do Canto e Castro Mascarenhas. *Diccionario español-portugués: El primero que se ha publicado con las voces . . . usadas en España y Americas españolas, en el lenguaje comun antiguo y moderno; las ciencias y artes de medicina, veterinaria, quimica, mineralojia, historia natural y botanica, comercio y nautica.* . . . 3 vols. Lisbon: Imprensa Nacional, 1864–66.

INDEX

abscess, 75, 114
acid, vegetable, 95
acrimony, 79
Afonso, Ignácio Caetano, 10
Africa, 4, 10–13, 45, 51, 65, 67, 76, 90;
coast of, 67, 76; east, 10; Europeans
in, 51; illness of, 65, 90, 100, 107; medicinal substances of, 13; population,
51; trees of, 84; west, 13
Africans, 3–6, 12–13, 51, 88–89, 91
água de Inglaterra, 93–94, 96
air: in Brazil, 3; as cause of disease,
25, 45, 52, 83–84, 86–88; fixed, 95;
mephitic, 83
alkali, 35, 97
Alvarenga, Silva, 32–33
America, 44, 63, 84–85; South, 6–8, 13
amputation, 128
Angola, 1, 3, 5, 9–10, 13, 31, 37, 42–43, 51,
88, 93; bloodletting in, 63; dysentery
in, 65, 107; education in, 38; fevers
of, 3, 24–25, 46, 62–63, 81; interior
of, 13, 51; people of, 13, 27; plants of,
84; public health in, 27; rain in, 83,
86–87; water in, 82–83
Angolans, 13, 51, 63, 84, 88–89, 91
animal economy, 80
anorexia, 107–8, 110, 123
antimony, 47, 92–93, 96, 115–16
antiscorbutic, 90
antiseptic, 50
antispasmodic, 8, 129
anxiety, 68, 74, 98–99
appetite, 123; lack of, 68, 71, 74
arsenic, 47, 106
artery, 69
Asclepiades of Bithynia, 78
asthenia, 80
astringents, 8, 116, 120

atony, 80
autopsy, 45
Azeredo, Francisco Pinto de, 11, 32–33,
36, 42
Azeredo, José Pinto de: in Angola/
Luanda, 3, 5, 9, 12–13, 37–38, 44, 51;
birth, 1, 32; death, 31, 42; early life
and education, 3, 14, 31–36; in Edinburgh, 1, 3, 11, 33–36; family, 32; historical significance of, 1–3, 12, 14–15,
42, 45; intellectual influences on, 1, 3,
5–6, 13, 15, 22–26, 33–34, 43–44, 49–
52; in Leiden, 3, 36; library, personal,
42, 44; in Lisbon, 31, 36, 40–42;
medical methodology, 1, 5, 45–50;
medical training, 1, 3, 33–35, 44–45;
as physician of the royal chamber,
40; in Rio de Janeiro, 3, 32–33, 36–37;
teachings, 4, 12, 15, 23–28, 37–38,
44. *See also* Azeredo, José Pinto de,
works of
Azeredo, José Pinto de, works of:
"Chemical Examinations of the
Atmosphere of Rio de Janeiro," 1, 15,
37, 43; "Clinical Observations," 39–
41, 44; "Essays on Some Maladies
of Angola," 1, 13, 15, 21, 24–25, 28, 31,
37, 39, 42, 44–45 "Introduction to the
Pathology of the Human Body," 35,
39–40, 44–45

Bacon, Francis, 48, 67, 79
Badenoch, James, 64
Baglivi, Gjuro (George), 27, 79
Bahia, Brazil, 6–8, 13, 63
Bajon, Bertrand, 129
Baker, George, 107
balsam, 84; catholic, 96
Bartholin, Thomas, 112

Index

dysentery, 24–25, 49, 65, 73–75, 81, 127; essay on, 107–21
dyspepsia, 111
dyspnea, 122, 125

earth (soil), 82, 115
edema, 74, 89, 110
Edinburgh, Scotland: city of, 3, 33, *34*, 35–36, 42; university of, 5, 33, *34*, 36, 47
effluvia, 88, 111, 115
emetic, 47, 92, 95–96, 104–6, 115–16, 118
empiricism, 2, 23–24, 45, 50, 64
England, 1, 11, 89
Enlightenment, vii, 1, 9, 12, 22–23, 26–27, 31, 43
entambe (indigenous Angolan mourning rituals), 89
epidemic, 81, 107, 111
exiles, 85. See also *degredados*
Europe, 1–3, 6, 11, 13, 33, 44, 47, 61, 84–85
evacuation, 46, 81, 95, 107–10, 112, 115–20
exanthema, 66

face, 46, 69, 76; inflamed, 49, 66, 68, 71; pale, 123; swollen, 130
fatigue, 125
fecal matter, 108, 111. *See also* feces
feces, 92, 107
fermentation, 46, 79, 112
Ferreira, Alexandre Rodrigues, 6–7
Ferreira, Luís Gomes, 6
fever, 9, 12–13, 25, 46, 63, 65; abatement of, 48, 66–67, 70, 76, 97, 105, 115; continuing/continuous, 48–49, 67, 92–93, 103; cure, 3, 9, 45, 47–48; definition, 66–67; inflammatory, 48–49, 66, 74, 80; intermittent, 39, 47, 49–50, 65, 104–6; mortal, 51, 70, 72, 91; nervous, 67, 80, 98; nosography of, 46–47; primary, 66, 48; remission, 66–71, 92–95, 98–99, 101–2, 123; remittent, 39, 47, 49–50, 67–103;

symptomatic, 48–49, 66–67; tropical, 46, 51
fevers, intermittent, essay on: cure, 104–6; definition, 66–67; history, 104; proximate cause, 104; remote causes, 104
fevers, remittent, essay on: cure, 91–103; definition, 66–67; history, 67–77; proximate cause, 78–81; remote causes, 81–91
fiber, 50, 76, 79–80, 90, 104, 114–15
flatulence, 74, 99, 108, 114
folk healing, 10, 88
France, 1, 15, 36
Franco, Francisco Mello, 46–48

Galen/Galenic medicine, 45, 47, 78
gangrene, 109, 111, 113–14
gas, 86–88, 108
Gaubius, Hieronymus David, 80, 125
Gilchrist, Ebenezer, 103
glands: parotid, 74; saliva, 90
gluttony, 90
Goa, India: city of, 10, 13; royal military hospital of, 4, 10
Gregory, James, 34
gum: ammoniac, 101; kino, 120
gums, 76

Haller, Albrecht von, 27, 80
Harvey, William, 78
headache, 68, 74, 97, 100, 103
heat, body, vii, 25, 68, 78, 90, 94, 97–98, 108, 111, 115
hemorrhage, 66, 77, 110
hemorrhoids, 110
hepatitis, 73, 114
Hewson, William, 79, 112
hiccups, 109
hip bath, 101, 119
Hippocrates, 36, 51, 64, 76–77
Hippocratic, 27, 45, 77
Hoffman, Friedrich, 44, 79, 89
Holy Office, 11. *See also* Inquisition, Portuguese

Index

Home, Francis, 34, 128
Hooke, Robert, 52
humorists, 26, 80
humors, 25, 79
Hunter, John (1728–1793), 34, 64–65, 107
Hunter, John (?–1809), 96
hydrocephalus, 75, 102
hygienism, 42
hysteria, 128

incision, 131
India, 4, 10, 13, 85
indigestion, 74, 90, 97
infirmity, 128
inflammation, 48–49, 66, 73–74, 114, 119–21, 127
Ingenhousz, Jan, 83
Inquisition, Portuguese, 1, 11
insomnia, 25, 90, 129
intestines, 89, 92–93, 96, 99, 104–5, 108–15, 117–20, 127–28
ipecacuanha (ipecac), 115, 118, 120
ivory, 43

jalapa (jalap), 14
James, powders of, 96
jasmine, 84
jaundice, 72
Jesuits, 13
João, Prince (Regent of Portugal), 8, 39–40, 61–62
juice, lemon, 95

Kant, Immanuel, 22–23
kola nut (cola nut), 85, 91
Kwanza River. *See* Cuanza River

lancet, 100
languor, 68, 74
laxative, 83, 95, 99, 106, 116, 118, 120
Leeuwenhoek, Antonie Philips van, 52
legs, symptoms in, 76, 102, 110, 124
Leiden, the Netherlands, 3, 5, 12, 36
Lemery, Nicolas, 79

lemonade, 97, 102
Lemos, Maximiano, 47
lethargy, 27, 69–70, 72, 99, 125–26
Lind, James, 64, 128
Linnaeus, Carl, 112
liquor, 89, 99
Lisbon: city of, 1, 3, 6–10, 12–13, 36–39, *41*, 42–43; royal military hospital of, 6, 40
liver, 46, 73, 89; inflammation of 73; obstruction of 73
logwood, 120
London, England, 11–12, 34, 36, 89
Luanda, Angola: city of, 5, 9, 12–13, 31, 37, 39, 43, 51, 82–87, 105; illness of (*mal de Luanda*), 85; royal hospital of, 38, 44
Lusitania, 62

Maddox, Isaac, 47
Maia, Emílio Joaquim da Silva, 31–33
Maianga, Angola, 82
malaria, 50
mal de Luanda, 85. *See also* scurvy
Malpighi, Marcello, 52
manna, 92, 101, 116
Maranhão, Brazil, 9
Maria I, Queen of Portugal (1777–1816), 2, 7–8, 10, 43, 51
Mello, Bento Bandeira de, 7
memory, loss of, 69
Mendes, Fernando, 11
mercury, 47, 50, 65, 101–2, 116–17, 130
metaphysics, 23, 40
miasma, 46, 86
microscope, 42, 45
milk, 93–94, 119; with quinine, 93
milongos, 88
Missengle, 82
mites, intestinal, 112
Monro, Alexander II, 34
Montpellier, France, 47
Morais, João David de, ix, 50
Morgagni, Giovanni Battista, 114
muscle tone, lack of, 75, 114

Index

Index

Index

Library of Congress Cataloging-in-Publication Data

Names: Azeredo, José Pinto de, 1763–1807, author. | Walker, Timothy Dale,
1963– , editor. | Cardoso, Adelino, editor. | Oliveira, António Braz de, editor. |
Marques, Manuel Silvério, 1946– , editor.
Title: Essays on some maladies of Angola (1799) / José Pinto de Azeredo;
translated by Stewart Lloyd-Jones; edited by Timothy D. Walker, Adelino
Cardoso, António Braz de Oliveira, and Manuel Silvério Marques.
Other titles: Ensaios sobre algumas enfermidades de Angola. English |
Classic histories from the Portuguese-speaking world in translation ; 2.
Description: Dartmouth, Massachusetts: Tagus Press at UMass Dartmouth,
[2016] | Series: Classic histories from the Portuguese-speaking world in
translation ; 2 | Includes bibliographical references and index.
Identifiers: LCCN 2015040144 (print) | LCCN 2015040808 (ebook) |
ISBN 9781933227696 (pbk.) | ISBN 9781933227702 (epub, mobi & pdf)
Subjects: MESH: Communicable Diseases—Angola—Essays.
Classification: LCC RA643 (print) | LCC RA643 (ebook) | NLM WZ 290 |
DDC 616.909673—dc23

LC record available at http://lccn.loc.gov/2015040144